ENDOMORPH
DIET FOR BEGINNERS

A 30 Day Meal Plan with Balanced and Delicious Recipes to Achieve Weight Loss, Boost Metabolism and Burn Fat

Kyla Miranda

Copyright© 2024 by Kyla Miranda

All rights reserved worldwide.

No part of this book may be reproduced or transmitted in any form or by any means, electronic or mechanical, including photo- copying, recording or by any information storage and retrieval system, without written permission from the publisher, except for the inclusion of brief quotations in a review.

Warning-Disclaimer

The purpose of this book is to educate and entertain. The author or publisher does not guarantee that anyone following the techniques, suggestions, tips, ideas, or strategies will become successful. The author and publisher shall have either liability or responsibility to anyone with respect to any loss or damage caused, or alleged to be caused, directly or indirectly by the information contained in this book.

Table of Contents

INTRODUCTION 6

CHAPTER 1: INTRODUCTION TO THE ENDOMORPH BODY TYPE 7

What is an Endomorph? 7
Overview of Body Types and Endomorph Characteristics 7
Common Challenges and Dietary Needs for Endomorphs 8
Benefits of a Tailored Diet for Endomorphs 9

CHAPTER 2: LIFESTYLE TIPS FOR ENDOMORPHS 11

CHAPTER 3: BREAKFAST RECIPES 15

Avocado & Spinach Power Omelet 15
Greek Yogurt Parfait with Nuts & Berries 16
Smoked Salmon & Asparagus Scramble 17
Almond Butter & Chia Seed Smoothie 18
Low-Carb Egg Muffins with Veggies 19
Protein Pancakes with Fresh Berries 20
Cottage Cheese & Cucumber Bowl 21
Coconut Flour Waffles 22
Cauliflower Hash Browns with Eggs 23
Broccoli & Cheese Frittata 24
Berry & Flaxseed Smoothie Bowl 25
Green Detox Smoothie 26
Scrambled Eggs with Kale & Cherry Tomatoes 27
Low-Carb Banana Protein Muffins 28
Veggie & Turkey Breakfast Wrap 29
Mushroom & Spinach Breakfast Casserole 30
Keto Cinnamon Chia Pudding 31
Zucchini & Bell Pepper Breakfast Hash 32
Salmon & Avocado Breakfast Bowl 33
Almond Flour Blueberry Muffins 34

CHAPTER 4: LUNCH RECIPES 35

Grilled Chicken & Quinoa Salad 35
Cauliflower Rice stir-fried with Shrimp 36
Spinach & Avocado Tuna Salad 37
Greek Chicken Salad Wrap 38
Turkey & Veggie Lettuce Wraps 39
Zucchini Noodles with Pesto & Cherry Tomatoes 40
Steak & Roasted Veggie Bowl 41
Sesame Salmon Salad 42
Cauliflower Crust Veggie Pizza 43
Grilled Halloumi & Arugula Salad 44
Baked Lemon Herb Cod with Spinach 45
Quinoa & Roasted Veggie Buddha Bowl 46
Thai Chicken Lettuce Cup 47

Chicken Caesar Salad with Kale 48
Blackened Shrimp & Cauliflower Grits 49
Mediterranean Veggie Bowl with Hummus 50
Low-Carb Turkey Avocado Wrap 51
Asian Ginger Chicken & Cabbage Slaw 52
Lemon Garlic Zoodles with Shredded Chicken 53
Low-Carb Taco Salad 54

CHAPTER 5: DINNER RECIPES **56**

Baked Salmon with Asparagus 56
Garlic & Herb Roasted Chicken with Brussels Sprouts 57
Zucchini Lasagna with Ground Turkey 58
Cauliflower Crust Margherita Pizza 59
Keto-Friendly Stuffed Bell Peppers 61
Beef & Broccoli Stir-Fry 62
Spaghetti Squash Bolognese 63
Seared Scallops with Zoodles 64
Grilled Shrimp with Cilantro Lime Cauliflower Rice 65
Low-Carb Turkey Meatloaf 66
Moroccan-Spiced Chicken with Spinach 67
Slow-Cooked Beef Stew with Veggies 68
Low-Carb Pork Chops with Garlic Mushrooms 70
Sheet Pan Salmon & Veggies 71
Grilled Veggie & Chicken Kebabs 72
Eggplant Parmesan Casserole 73
Thai Basil Chicken Stir-Fry 74
Lemon Pepper Tilapia with Steamed Greens 75
Low-Carb Lamb & Vegetable Curry 76
Spicy Cauliflower & Chicken Skillet 77

CHAPTER 6: SNACKS AND SIDES **79**

Guacamole & Veggie Sticks 79
Baked Zucchini Fries 80
Deviled Eggs with Avocado 81
Greek Yogurt Ranch Dip with Cucumbers 82
Low-Carb Cheese & Meat Platter 83
Spicy Roasted Chickpeas 84
Broccoli Cheddar Bites 85
Almond-Crusted Mozzarella Sticks 86
Keto Cauliflower Hummus 87
Celery Sticks with Nut Butter 88
Bell Pepper Nachos with Ground Turkey 89
Stuffed Mushrooms with Spinach & Feta 90
Lemon & Garlic Roasted Asparagus 91
Cucumber & Avocado Rolls 92
Mini Caprese Salad Skewers 93
Baked Brussels Sprouts Chips 94
Spiced Cauliflower Popcorn 95

Turkey & Cheese Roll-Ups 96
Keto-Friendly Trail Mix 97
Sautéed Garlic Green Beans 98

CHAPTER 7: DESSERT RECIPES 99
Almond Flour Chocolate Chip Cookies 99
Keto Vanilla Mug Cake 100
Low-Carb Cheesecake Bites 101
Chocolate Avocado Mousse 102
Keto Coconut Macaroons 103
Chia Seed Pudding with Berries 104
Keto Almond Butter Fudge 105
Strawberry & Cream Keto Popsicles 106
Coconut Flour Brownies 107
Lemon Coconut Energy Balls 108
Chocolate Protein Truffles 109
Pumpkin Spice Fat Bombs 110
Low-Carb Cinnamon Apple Crisp 111
Coconut Panna Cotta 112
Peanut Butter & Chocolate Keto Cup 113
Almond Butter Blondies 114
Mocha Coconut Keto Ice Cream 115

30 DAYS MEAL PLAN 116

INTRODUCTION

Welcome to "Endomorph Diet for Beginners," your complete guide to understanding and embracing the endomorph body type's specific nutritional requirements. Whether you are new to the concept of body types or have tried unsuccessfully to control your weight, this book will give you the knowledge, skills, and recipes you need to live a healthy lifestyle that is customized particularly to your genetic blueprint.

In the early 20th century, psychologist William Sheldon defined three major body types: endomorphs, ectomorphs, and mesomorphs. Endomorphs have a fuller form and typically struggle with weight gain owing to their body's propensity to accumulate fat. However, with the correct diet and lifestyle changes, endomorphs may successfully control their weight and stay healthy.

This book will review the fundamental concepts of the endomorph diet, which stresses a balanced intake of carbohydrates, proteins, and fats. It emphasizes explicitly carbohydrate management and increasing protein and fiber consumption. Understanding which foods to consume and which to avoid allows you to develop a meal plan that meets your body's demands without feeling deprived.

In "Endomorph Diet for Beginners, "you'll discover not just theoretical information but also practical guidance. This book features tasty, easy-to-follow recipes that meet your nutritional demands. In addition, it provides insights into effective workout techniques that match nutritional modifications, allowing you to attain the most significant potential outcomes.

Whether you want to lose weight, increase your fitness, or live a better lifestyle, this book will confidently guide you. Let's go on this transformational journey together, learning to tailor your food to your endomorphic body and embrace a healthier, happier self.

CHAPTER 1: INTRODUCTION TO THE ENDOMORPH BODY TYPE

What is an Endomorph?

William Sheldon, a psychologist, developed the concept of body types, or somatotypes, in the early twentieth century. He classified bodies into three types based on appearance and characteristics: ectomorphs, mesomorphs, and endomorphs. Each kind has unique traits and metabolic consequences, which may help people choose the most successful diet and exercise methods.

Among them, the endomorph body type is defined by a sturdy, frequently spherical shape and a tendency to accumulate body fat. Endomorphs often have a soft, curvier physique, broader hips, and a lot of body mass. This body type might simplify muscle building, but fat loss is more difficult due to a slower metabolism.

Understanding the body's demands may help endomorphs achieve their health and fitness objectives. Effective treatment often requires a personalized strategy for food and exercise, emphasizing balancing macronutrient consumption and including both aerobic and strength training activities to maximize metabolism and muscle mass.

Recognizing these qualities might help endomorphs make more educated health choices, enabling them to work with rather than against their bodies.

Overview of Body Types and Endomorph Characteristics

Understanding body types is essential for adapting nutrition, exercise, and lifestyle choices to meet individual demands efficiently. Each kind has unique characteristics and metabolic habits that affect how the body consumes food and reacts to physical activity.

1. Ectomorphs

Ectomorphs are often defined by their lean and lengthy bodies. They have little body fat and muscle and generally struggle to acquire weight due to a high metabolic rate. This body type excels in tasks that require endurance and agility but may fail to gain significant muscle mass.

2. Mesomorphs

Mesomorphs have a naturally athletic build, well-defined muscles, a robust frame, and an efficient metabolism. This body type gains and loses weight reasonably quickly and benefits from a balanced approach to strength and cardiovascular training. Mesomorphs may adapt to various sports and excel at activities requiring power and speed.

3. Endomorphs

Endomorphs have a more extensive form and an increased capacity to store body fat. They usually have a rounder shape, with fat concentrated around the abdomen. Endomorphs may have difficulty losing weight due to their slower metabolism, which conserves energy more efficiently than other body types.

Common Challenges and Dietary Needs for Endomorphs

Managing their weight and general health presents some typical difficulties for endomorphs. Their unique body composition and metabolism rate make them prone to several problems, especially in a modern world with standard high-calorie diets and inactive lives. The first step in developing workable plans to overcome these difficulties is knowledge.

Common Challenges for Endomorphs:

Weight gain Susceptibility: Endomorphs acquire weight quickly owing to their slower metabolism. This might make it harder to reduce weight after gaining weight, as it requires more work than other body types.

Energy variations: Because of their insulin sensitivity, endomorphs may suffer more variations in energy levels throughout the Day. These fluctuations frequently result in feelings of fatigue, especially following carbohydrate-rich meals.

Difficulty in Fat Loss: Even with a calorie deficit, endomorphs may discover that losing fat takes longer. Their bodies are predisposed to accumulate fat, a backup energy source.

Food cravings: Insulin resistance can cause increased cravings for sugary or carbohydrate-rich meals, making diet adherence more difficult.

Dietary Needs for Endomorphs:

To effectively manage these problems, endomorphs must follow a nutritional plan that regulates their metabolism and promotes a better body composition. Key features of this diet include:

Lower Carbohydrate Intake: Reducing the amount of carbohydrates consumed, particularly refined sugars and starches, can help reduce insulin spikes and better control energy levels. Instead, eating complex carbs with a low glycemic index, such as vegetables, whole grains, and legumes, is advantageous.

Higher Protein Consumption: Consuming more protein can improve satiety, assist in maintaining muscle mass, and raise metabolic rate. Endomorphs rely on proteins for muscle growth since they do not cause the fast insulin response that carbohydrates do.

Healthy Fats: Fats are necessary for hormonal balance and can assist in maintaining sensations of fullness. Avocados, almonds, seeds, and fatty fish promote satiety while providing consistent energy release.

Fiber-Rich Foods: High-fiber foods are essential for an endomorph diet since they slow digestion, promote gut health, and increase satiety. Vegetables, fruits, whole grains, and legumes should be staples in your diet.

Regular, Balanced Meals: Eating at regular intervals can help prevent large energy drops and cravings, which can contribute to overeating. It's also a good idea to incorporate a range of foods to ensure that all nutrients are properly eaten.

Hydration: Staying hydrated is essential for all body types, especially for endomorphs needing assistance with metabolism and digestion.

Benefits of a Tailored Diet for Endomorphs

Adopting a diet adapted to the unique demands of endomorphs can provide considerable benefits beyond weight management. Endomorphs can improve their health, energy levels, and general quality of life by tailoring their dietary choices to their specific metabolic and physiological traits. Here are some of the main advantages of a customized diet for endomorphs:

Increased Metabolic Efficiency: Endomorphs can regulate their sluggish metabolism with a diet low in carbs and high in protein and healthy fats. This nutritional balance helps to maintain blood sugar levels, lowering the chance of insulin spikes and crashes, which can alter body weight and mood.

Improved Weight Management: Endomorphs might benefit from a diet that reduces simple carbs while boosting fiber and protein intake. This method minimizes the body's propensity to retain fat and improves its capacity to use fat as a fuel source, resulting in progressive and consistent weight reduction.

Increased Energy: By controlling carbohydrate consumption and focusing on foods that promote sustained energy release, endomorphs can experience fewer energy dips throughout the day. This consistent energy level can boost focus, productivity, and mood.

Reduced Risk of Chronic Diseases: Endomorphs are more likely to develop type 2 diabetes, cardiovascular disease, and metabolic syndrome. A diet customized to their specific requirements can help reduce these risks by improving metabolic health, lowering body fat, and increasing cardiovascular function.

Better Hormone Balance: Proper diet is crucial for hormonal balance. Endomorphs require a well-balanced diet of fats and proteins to maintain appropriate levels of hormones such as insulin and leptin, which regulate hunger, metabolism, and fat accumulation.

Greater Physical Performance: Endomorphs can enhance their muscular build and strength by increasing their protein intake and eating more nutrient-dense meals. This not only aids in weight management but also improves physical performance, making exercise more accessible and more effective.

Increased Satiety and Decreased Cravings: A well-planned diet with enough fiber and protein can help endomorphs feel fuller for extended periods, lowering the risk of overeating. This can also help reduce cravings for harmful foods, making sticking to a balanced eating plan simpler.

Personalization and adaptability: A personalized diet considers each individual's unique needs, tastes, and lifestyle. This tailored approach improves the diet's effectiveness and makes it more pleasurable and sustainable in the long run.

CHAPTER 2: LIFESTYLE TIPS FOR ENDOMORPHS

The Importance of Exercise for Endomorphs

Diet alone can only go you so far. Endomorphs naturally store fat more efficiently and have a slower metabolism, requiring the correct workout routine to maximize fat reduction, build lean muscle, and improve metabolic health. While all types of exercise are helpful, strength training and High-Intensity Interval Training (HIIT) are efficient for endomorphs. Let's examine why different kinds of exercise are essential and how they may help you achieve an attractive body.

1. Strength Training

Endomorphs often have a slower metabolism and burn fewer calories at rest than other body types. What's the solution? Develop more muscle. Muscle tissue is metabolically active, which means it needs more energy (calories) to function than fat tissue. This implies that the more muscle you make, the more calories you burn, even if you're simply sitting on a couch.

Benefits of Strength Training

Lifting weights increases your resting metabolic rate (RMR), the number of calories your body burns while at rest. This metabolic increase is significant for endomorphs, who usually burn fewer calories.

Improved body Composition: Strength training can help you alter your physique by burning fat and building muscular mass. This improves your physical look and increases your body's ability to burn calories.

Reduced Insulin Sensitivity: Endomorphs frequently struggle with insulin sensitivity, making it challenging to reduce weight. Strength training increases insulin sensitivity, allowing your body to control blood sugar levels better and reduce fat accumulation.

Critical Exercises to Focus On

Prioritize compound workouts such as squats, deadlifts, bench presses, and rows. These movements work numerous muscle groups, burning more calories and increasing functional strength.

Resistance Training: Use free weights, resistance bands, or bodyweight exercises. Aim for three to four sessions per week, each concentrating on a different muscle area.

Progressive Overload: To make steady progress, progressively increase the weight or resistance you utilize. This promotes muscular development and keeps your metabolism active.

2. High-Intensity Interval Training (HIIT)

Endomorphs frequently find that standard steady-state exercise (such as running consistently) cannot break through weight reduction plateaus. They are introducing High-Intensity Interval Training (HIIT), a time-saving and effective technique for burning calories, increasing cardiovascular fitness, and targeting stubborn fat.

Why HIIT Works for Endomorphs:

Afterburn Effect (EPOC): HIIT exercises make an "afterburn" effect, scientifically recognized as excess post-exercise oxygen consumption. This implies that your body will continue to burn calories at a greater rate even after your workout. Endomorphs who want to lose weight will benefit the most from this increased calorie burn.

Efficient Fat Burning: HIIT workouts alternate between brief bursts of intense exertion followed by rest or low-intensity activity. This method helps you burn more fat in less time than standard cardio routines.

Improved Cardiovascular Health: HIIT not only promotes weight reduction but also improves heart health, endurance, and general stamina. This is especially essential for endomorphs, more likely to develop metabolic disorders like high blood pressure or insulin resistance.

How to Incorporate HIIT:

Choose your workout: HIIT may be performed with nearly any workout, including jumping jacks, sprints, cycling, burpees, and kettlebell swings. The goal is to push oneself to a high level during the "work" intervals.

Structure your workout: A standard HIIT structure consists of 20 seconds of challenging activity followed by 10 seconds of recovery, done eight times. However, you may tailor your intervals to your fitness level, such as 30 seconds of effort and 30 seconds of rest.

Begin with 2-3 HIIT workouts each week, allowing your body to adjust and recover. Alternate between HIIT and strength training days for a well-rounded exercise program.

3. The Synergy of Strength Training and HIIT

Strength training and HIIT make a compelling pair for endomorphs. They provide muscle-building and fat-burning advantages, helping reduce body fat and reshape the body by improving muscle definition and strength.

Increased Calorie Burn: Strength training develops muscle, whereas HIIT burns fat. Together, they form a calorie-burning powerhouse that aids endomorphs in overcoming their unique metabolic problems.

Improved Hormonal Balance: Both forms of exercise assist in balancing critical hormones like insulin and cortisol, which might otherwise cause fat accumulation in endomorphs.

Enhanced Mood and Energy Levels: Regular exercise produces endorphins, decreases stress, and increases energy levels, which can help endomorphs stick to their diet and fitness regimens with more excellent drive and consistency.

4. Tips for Getting Started

Start Slowly: If you're new to fitness, begin with strength training and HIIT with lesser weights and shorter periods. Gradually raise the intensity as your fitness increases.

Listen to your body. Specific workouts may be more difficult for endomorphs, especially if they are overweight. Focus on the appropriate forms to avoid injuries and alter the intensity as needed.

Make exercise a regular ingredient of your schedule. Aim for a combination of strength and HIIT workouts, with active recovery days in between.

5. Creating a Balanced Exercise Plan

Endomorphs should work out 4-5 days per week, alternating between cardio, weight training, and flexibility activities. Here's an example of a weekly routine:

Day 1: 30 minutes of steady-state cardio (e.g., cycling or brisk walking) + 20 minutes of full-body strength training

Day 2: HIIT workout (20-30 minutes) + core exercises (planks, Russian twists)

Day 3: Rest day or active recovery

Day 4: Upper body strength training (push-ups, dumbbell rows, bicep curls)

Day 5: 40 minutes of cardio (mix of steady-state and interval training)

Day 6: Lower body strength training (squats, lunges, leg presses)

Day 7: Flexibility and mobility work (yoga or Pilates)

CHAPTER 3: BREAKFAST RECIPES

Avocado & Spinach Power Omelet

Prep Time: 10 minutes

Cook Time: 5 minutes

Serving: 1

Ingredients:

- 2 large eggs
- 1 tbsp olive oil
- 1/2 avocado, peeled and sliced
- 1 cup of fresh spinach leaves
- 1/4 cup of feta cheese, crumbled
- Salt and pepper to taste
- Optional garnish: fresh parsley or chives

Instructions:

1. In a mixing bowl, whisk the eggs until well combined. Season with salt and pepper.
2. Heat the olive oil in a nonstick skillet over medium heat. Sauté the spinach in the pan until barely wilted, about 1-2 minutes.
3. Pour the eggs over the spinach and simmer for approximately 2 minutes or until they begin to set on the bottom and sides.
4. Gently arrange the avocado slices and feta cheese on one half of the omelet.
5. Carefully fold the remaining half of the omelet over the filled side. Cook for 1-2 more to allow the feta to melt gently.
6. Place the omelet on a platter and garnish with parsley or chives if desired.

Nutrition Information:

Calories: 400 Protein: 18 g Fat: 34 g Carbohydrates: 8 g Fiber: 5 g Sugar: 2 g

Greek Yogurt Parfait with Nuts & Berries

Prep Time: 5 minutes

Cook Time: 0 minutes

Serving: 1

Ingredients:

- 1 cup of Greek yogurt (full-fat)
- 1/4 cup of mixed berries
- 1/4 cup of mixed nuts (almonds, walnuts, pecans), roughly chopped
- 1 tbsp chia seeds
- 1 tsp honey (optional)

Instructions:

1. In a serving glass or bowl, place half of the Greek yogurt on the bottom.
2. Add a layer of mixed berries, chopped almonds, and half of the chia seeds.
3. Repeat layering with the remaining yogurt, berries, almonds, and chia seeds. If desired, drizzle the top with honey to add sweetness.
4. Serve immediately.

Nutrition Information:

Calories: 320 Protein: 20 g Fat: 20 g Carbohydrates: 18 g Fiber: 4 g Sugar: 10 g

Smoked Salmon & Asparagus Scramble

Prep Time: 10 minutes

Cook Time: 8 minutes

Serving: 1

Ingredients:

- 2 large eggs
- 1/2 tbsp olive oil
- 100 grams smoked salmon, chopped
- 5 asparagus spears, trimmed and cut into 1-inch pieces
- 2 tbsp cream cheese
- Salt and pepper to taste
- Optional: 1 tbsp chopped dill or chives for garnish

Instructions:

1. In a mixing bowl, beat the eggs and season with salt and pepper. Set aside.
2. Heat the olive oil in a nonstick skillet over medium heat. Sauté the asparagus pieces for 3-4 minutes, until tender yet still crisp.
3. Reduce the heat and add the chopped smoked salmon to the skillet, stirring for approximately 1 minute to warm it.
4. Pour the beaten eggs onto the fish and asparagus. Let the eggs set slightly around the edges, then gently whisk in the salmon and asparagus.
5. Add the cream cheese to the scramble when the eggs are almost set but still somewhat runny. Cook for another minute, letting the cream cheese melt into the scramble.
6. Remove from the heat, sprinkle with dill or chives if desired, and serve immediately.

Nutrition Information:

Calories: 400 Protein: 25 g Fat: 30 g Carbohydrates: 5 g Fiber: 1 g Sugar: 2 g

Almond Butter & Chia Seed Smoothie

Prep Time: 5 minutes

Cook Time: 0 minutes

Serving: 1

Ingredients:

- 1 cup of unsweetened almond milk
- 1 banana, sliced
- 2 tbsp almond butter
- 1 tbsp chia seeds
- 1/2 tsp vanilla extract
- Ice cubes (optional)

Instructions:

1. Combine the almond milk, sliced banana, almond butter, chia seeds, and vanilla extract in a blender.
2. Add a handful of ice cubes if you want your smoothie colder and thicker.
3. Blend on high until completely smooth and creamy.
4. Pour into a glass and serve immediately.

Nutrition Information:

Calories: 350 Protein: 10 g Fat: 22 g Carbohydrates: 28 g Fiber: 7 g Sugar: 12 g

Low-Carb Egg Muffins with Veggies

Prep Time: 15 minutes

Cook Time: 20 minutes

Serving: 6 muffins

Ingredients:

- 6 large eggs
- 1/4 cup of milk (any kind)
- 1/2 cup of chopped bell peppers
- 1/2 cup of chopped broccoli
- 1/4 cup of chopped onion
- 1/2 cup of shredded cheese
- Salt and pepper to taste
- Non-stick cooking spray or olive oil for greasing

Instructions:

1. Preheat the oven to 375° Fahrenheit (190° Celsius). Grease a muffin pan with nonstick spray or a thin layer of olive oil.
2. In a large mixing bowl, whisk together the eggs and milk. Season with salt and pepper.
3. Combine the chopped bell peppers, broccoli, onion, and shredded cheese (if using).
4. Evenly spread the egg and veggie mixture into the muffin cups. Each cup should be approximately three-quarters full.
5. Bake in the oven for 20 minutes or until the tops are hard to the touch and the eggs are fully cooked.
6. Cool for a few minutes before removing it from the muffin tray.
7. Serve warm.

Nutrition Information:

Calories (per muffin): 120 Protein: 9 g Fat: 8 g Carbohydrates: 3 g Fiber: 1 g Sugar: 2 g

Protein Pancakes with Fresh Berries

Prep Time: 10 minutes

Cook Time: 10 minutes

Serving: 2

Ingredients:

- 1/2 cup of oat flour
- 1/2 cup of cottage cheese
- 2 large eggs
- 1/4 cup of milk (any kind)
- 1 scoop protein powder (vanilla or unflavored)
- 1/2 tsp baking powder
- 1/2 tsp vanilla extract
- Pinch of salt
- Cooking spray or butter for greasing
- 1 cup of fresh berries
- Optional: Sugar-free maple syrup or honey for serving

Instructions:

1. Mix the oat flour, cottage cheese, eggs, milk, protein powder, baking powder, vanilla extract, and salt in a blender. Blend until smooth.
2. Heat a nonstick pan over medium heat and gently coat with cooking spray or a little butter.
3. Pour roughly 1/4 cup of batter into each pancake in the heated skillet. Cook for 2-3 minutes on one side until bubbles form and the edges dry.
4. Flip the pancakes and heat for another 2-3 minutes or until golden brown and thoroughly done.
5. If preferred, serve the pancakes warm, with fresh berries and a sprinkle of sugar-free maple syrup or honey.

Nutrition Information:

Calories (per serving): 350 Protein: 25 g Fat: 10 g Carbohydrates: 34 g Fiber: 5 g Sugar: 8 g

Cottage Cheese & Cucumber Bowl

Prep Time: 5 minutes

Cook Time: 0 minutes

Serving: 1

Ingredients:

- 1 cup of cottage cheese
- 1 small cucumber, diced
- 1/2 red bell pepper, diced
- 2 tbsp chopped red onion
- 1 tbsp lemon juice
- 1 tbsp fresh dill, chopped
- Salt and pepper to taste
- Optional: 1 tbsp olive oil for extra richness

Instructions:

1. Add cottage cheese, chopped cucumber, red bell pepper, and red onion in a bowl.
2. Drizzle with lemon juice and, if desired, olive oil. Stir until well combined.
3. Season with salt and pepper. Garnish with fresh dill.
4. Serve immediately, or chill in the refrigerator for 30 minutes to intensify the flavors.

Nutrition Information:

Calories: 200 Protein: 25 g Fat: 5 g Carbohydrates: 10 g Fiber: 2 g Sugar: 8 g

Coconut Flour Waffles

Prep Time: 10 minutes

Cook Time: 15 minutes

Serving: 2

Ingredients:

- 1/2 cup of coconut flour
- 1 tsp baking powder
- 1/4 tsp salt
- 4 large eggs
- 1/4 cup of milk (almond milk for a dairy-free option)
- 2 tbsp coconut oil, melted
- 1 tbsp honey or sweetener of choice
- 1/2 tsp vanilla extract
- Cooking spray or additional coconut oil for greasing the waffle iron

Instructions:

1. Combine the coconut flour, baking powder, and salt in a large bowl.
2. In a separate bowl, whisk the eggs, then add the milk, melted coconut oil, honey, and vanilla extract.
3. Combine the wet and dry ingredients and whisk until the batter is smooth.
4. Preheat the waffle iron and coat it with cooking spray or coconut oil. Pour just enough batter into the waffle iron to cover the grid.
5. Close the iron and cook according to the manufacturer's directions, generally around 5 minutes, until the waffle is golden and crisp.
6. Carefully remove the waffle, then repeat with the remaining batter.
7. Serve hot with your desired toppings.

Nutrition Information:

Calories (per serving): 280 Protein: 12 g Fat: 18 g Carbohydrates: 16 g Fiber: 10 g Sugar: 4 g

Cauliflower Hash Browns with Eggs

Prep Time: 15 minutes

Cook Time: 10 minutes

Serving: 2

Ingredients:

- 2 cups of cauliflower, grated
- 1 small onion, finely chopped
- 1 garlic clove, minced
- 2 large eggs
- 1/4 cup of almond flour
- Salt and pepper to taste
- 2 tbsp olive oil
- 4 eggs (for frying)
- Optional: chopped parsley or chives for garnish

Instructions:

1. Add grated cauliflower, chopped onion, minced garlic, two beaten eggs, and almond flour in a large mixing bowl. Season with salt and pepper, and stir until thoroughly blended.
2. In a large skillet, heat olive oil over medium heat.
3. Scoop a large spoonful of cauliflower mixture into the skillet and flatten to make a hash brown shape. Cook for 3-4 minutes per side until golden brown and crispy.
4. Remove the hash browns and put them aside. Reduce the heat to low and fry the remaining four eggs until they are cooked to your liking.
5. Top the hash browns with fried eggs and sprinkle with parsley or chives if desired.

Nutrition Information:

Calories (per serving): 320 Protein: 18 g Fat: 24 g Carbohydrates: 10 g Fiber: 4 g Sugar: 3 g

Broccoli & Cheese Frittata

Prep Time: 10 minutes

Cook Time: 20 minutes

Serving: 4

Ingredients:

- 6 large eggs
- 1/2 cup of milk
- 2 cups of broccoli florets, lightly steamed
- 1 cup of shredded cheddar cheese
- 1/2 onion, finely diced
- 2 tbsp olive oil
- Salt and pepper to taste
- Optional: 1/4 tsp nutmeg or paprika for added flavor

Instructions:

1. Preheat the oven to 375° Fahrenheit (190° Celsius).
2. Combine the eggs, milk, salt, and pepper in a large bowl.
3. Heat the olive oil in an oven-safe skillet over medium heat. Sauté the chopped onion until transparent, about 3-4 minutes.
4. Stir the steamed broccoli into the skillet.
5. Pour the egg mixture onto the broccoli and onions. Sprinkle the shredded cheese evenly over top.
6. Cook on the heat for about 5 minutes or until the edges are firm.
7. Place the pan in the oven for 15 minutes until the middle is set and the top is gently brown.
8. Remove from the oven, allow it to cool slightly, and then slice into wedges.

Nutrition Information:

Calories (per serving): 300 Protein: 20 g Fat: 22 g Carbohydrates: 8 g Fiber: 2 g Sugar: 3 g

Berry & Flaxseed Smoothie Bowl

Prep Time: 5 minutes

Cook Time: 0 minutes

Serving: 1

Ingredients:

- 1 cup of frozen mixed berries (blueberries, strawberries, raspberries)
- 1 banana
- 1/2 cup of Greek yogurt (full-fat)
- 1/4 cup of almond milk
- 1 tbsp flaxseed, ground
- Toppings: Additional berries, a sprinkle of granola, coconut flakes, chia seeds

Instructions:

1. Mix frozen berries, bananas, Greek yogurt, and almond milk in a blender. Blend until smooth.
2. Add the ground flaxseed and mix quickly to combine. Pour the smoothie into a bowl.
3. If preferred, add more berries, granola, coconut flakes, and chia seeds.
4. Serve immediately.

Nutrition Information:

Calories: 350 Protein: 15 g Fat: 7 g Carbohydrates: 55 g Fiber: 10 g Sugar: 30 g

Green Detox Smoothie

Prep Time: 5 minutes

Cook Time: 0 minutes

Serving: 1

Ingredients:

- 1 cup of fresh spinach leaves
- 1 small cucumber, peeled and chopped
- 1 green apple, cored and chopped
- 1/2 banana
- 1 tbsp fresh ginger, grated
- 1 tbsp lemon juice
- 1/2 cup of water or coconut water
- Ice cubes (optional)

Instructions:

1. Combine spinach, cucumber, green apple, banana, and grated ginger in a blender.
2. Combine lemon juice and water. If you want your smoothie colder and thicker, add ice cubes.
3. Blend at high speeds until smooth and creamy.
4. Pour into a glass and serve immediately.

Nutrition Information:

Calories: 180 Protein: 2 g Fat: 0.5 g Carbohydrates: 44 g Fiber: 6 g Sugar: 28 g

Scrambled Eggs with Kale & Cherry Tomatoes

Prep Time: 5 minutes

Cook Time: 10 minutes

Serving: 1

Ingredients:

- 2 large eggs
- 1 tbsp milk (optional for fluffier eggs)
- 1 cup of kale, washed and roughly chopped
- 1/2 cup of cherry tomatoes, halved
- 1 tbsp olive oil
- Salt and pepper to taste
- Optional: 1 tbsp grated Parmesan or nutritional yeast for a cheesy flavor

Instructions:

1. In a bowl, combine the eggs, milk (if using), and a touch of salt and pepper.
2. Heat the olive oil in a nonstick skillet over medium heat. Sauté the kale for 2-3 minutes until it begins to wilt.
3. Cook for 2 minutes or until the cherry tomatoes have softened somewhat.
4. Pour the egg mixture onto the greens and tomatoes. Allow them to remain for approximately a minute without stirring, then use a spatula to gently scramble the eggs until they are softly set and somewhat runny.
5. If preferred, sprinkle with Parmesan or nutritional yeast. Serve immediately.

Nutrition Information:

Calories: 300 Protein: 18 g Fat: 23 g Carbohydrates: 7 g Fiber: 2 g Sugar: 3 g

Low-Carb Banana Protein Muffins

Prep Time: 15 minutes

Cook Time: 20 minutes

Serving: 12 muffins

Ingredients:

- 2 medium ripe bananas, mashed
- 2 cups of almond flour
- 1/4 cup of vanilla protein powder
- 1/4 cup of erythritol (or another sugar substitute)
- 1 tsp baking powder
- 1/2 tsp baking soda
- 1/4 tsp salt
- 3 large eggs
- 1/4 cup of unsweetened almond milk
- 1/4 cup of coconut oil, melted
- 1 tsp vanilla extract

Instructions:

1. Preheat the oven to 350°F (175° C). Line a muffin tray with paper liners or spray with cooking spray.
2. Add almond flour, protein powder, erythritol, baking powder, soda, and salt to a large mixing bowl.
3. Combine the mashed bananas, eggs, almond milk, melted coconut oil, and vanilla extract in another bowl.
4. Mix the wet ingredients into the dry ingredients until just mixed.
5. Divide the mixture evenly among the muffin cups, filling them approximately 3/4 full.
6. Bake in a preheated oven for 18-20 minutes or until a toothpick inserted in the center of each muffin comes out clean.
7. Let the muffins cool in the pan for 5 minutes before transferring to a wire rack to finish cooling.

Nutrition Information:

Calories (per muffin): 180 Protein: 7 g Fat: 14 g Carbohydrates: 8 g Fiber: 3 g Sugar: 2 g

Veggie & Turkey Breakfast Wrap

Prep Time: 10 minutes

Cook Time: 5 minutes

Serving: 1

Ingredients:

- 1 large whole wheat or low-carb tortilla
- 3 ounces sliced turkey breast
- 1/2 cup of spinach leaves, washed
- 1/4 cup of grated carrot
- 2 tbsp hummus
- 1/4 avocado, sliced
- Salt and pepper to taste
- Optional: 1 tbsp salsa or Greek yogurt for topping

Instructions:

1. Place the tortilla flat on a clean surface. Spread the hummus evenly on the tortilla.
2. Spread the spinach leaves, chopped carrot, and avocado slices over the hummus.
3. Place the sliced turkey breast on top of the veggies. Season with salt and pepper.
4. Carefully roll the tortilla into a wrap, tucking in the sides to retain the fillings.
5. If preferred, prepare a nonstick pan over medium heat and lightly toast the wrap for 2-3 minutes on each side to warm the turkey and crisp the tortilla.
6. Slice in half and serve immediately, topped with salsa or Greek yogurt if desired.

Nutrition Information:

Calories: 350 Protein: 25 g Fat: 15 g Carbohydrates: 27 g Fiber: 6 g Sugar: 3 g

Mushroom & Spinach Breakfast Casserole

Prep Time: 15 minutes

Cook Time: 30 minutes

Serving: 6

Ingredients:

- 8 large eggs
- 1/2 cup of milk
- 2 cups of fresh spinach, roughly chopped
- 1 cup of mushrooms, sliced
- 1/2 onion, diced
- 1 cup of shredded cheddar cheese
- 2 tbsp olive oil
- Salt and pepper to taste
- Optional: 1/4 tsp nutmeg or garlic powder for extra flavor

Instructions:

1. Preheat the oven to 350°F (175° C). Grease a 9x13-inch baking dish with olive oil or cooking spray.
2. In a large skillet, heat olive oil over medium heat. Sauté the onions and mushrooms until they are transparent and the mushrooms have shed their moisture, which should take 5-7 minutes.
3. Cook the spinach in the pan for about 2 minutes or until it has wilted. Remove from heat.
4. Whisk the eggs, milk, salt, pepper, and other spices in a large mixing bowl. Add the cooked veggies and half of the cheese.
5. Pour the mixture into the prepared baking dish and top with the remaining cheese.
6. Bake for 25-30 minutes until the eggs are cooked and the top is gently brown.
7. Allow it to cool for a few minutes before slicing and serving.

Nutrition Information:

Calories (per serving): 220 Protein: 15 g Fat: 16 g Carbohydrates: 4 g Fiber: 1 g Sugar: 2 g

Keto Cinnamon Chia Pudding

Prep Time: 5 minutes

Cook Time: 0 minutes

Serving: 2

Ingredients:

- 1/4 cup of chia seeds
- 1 cup of unsweetened almond milk
- 1/2 cup of heavy cream
- 2 tbsp erythritol
- 1 tsp ground cinnamon
- 1/2 tsp vanilla extract
- Optional toppings: a sprinkle of nutmeg, toasted coconut, or sliced almonds

Instructions:

1. Add chia seeds, almond milk, heavy cream, erythritol, cinnamon, and vanilla extract in a bowl.
2. Whisk everything together until well blended.
3. Cover the bowl and refrigerate for at least 4 hours, or overnight, until the chia seeds have absorbed the liquid and the pudding is thick.
4. Once the pudding has set, whisk it to break up any clumps. If it is too thick, add more almond milk until it reaches the required consistency.
5. If preferred, serve chilled, garnished with nutmeg, toasted coconut, or sliced almonds.

Nutrition Information:

Calories: 310 Protein: 4 g Fat: 29 g Carbohydrates: 8 g Fiber: 6 g Sugar: 1 g

Zucchini & Bell Pepper Breakfast Hash

Prep Time: 10 minutes

Cook Time: 20 minutes

Serving: 2

Ingredients:

- 1 medium zucchini, diced
- 1 red bell pepper, diced
- 1 yellow bell pepper, diced
- 1 onion, diced
- 2 garlic cloves, minced
- 4 eggs
- 2 tbsp olive oil
- Salt and pepper to taste
- Optional: chopped fresh herbs like parsley or chives for garnish

Instructions:

1. In a large skillet, heat olive oil over medium heat.
2. Sauté the diced onion and garlic in the pan for approximately 5 minutes or until the onions become translucent.
3. Add the diced zucchini and bell peppers to the skillet. Season with salt and pepper. Cook for approximately 10-15 minutes, stirring periodically, until the veggies are soft and gently browned.
4. Make four wells in the hash and break an egg into each one. Cover the skillet and heat until the eggs are cooked to your taste, around 4-5 minutes for soft yolks.
5. Remove from the heat, sprinkle with fresh herbs if desired, and serve immediately.

Nutrition Information:

Calories (per serving): 320 Protein: 16 g Fat: 22 g Carbohydrates: 14 g Fiber: 3 g Sugar: 8 g

Salmon & Avocado Breakfast Bowl

Prep Time: 10 minutes

Cook Time: 5 minutes

Serving: 1

Ingredients:

- 4 oz smoked salmon
- 1 ripe avocado, sliced
- 1/2 cup of cooked quinoa
- 1 handful of arugula or baby spinach
- 1 small cucumber, sliced
- 1 tbsp capers
- 1/4 red onion, thinly sliced
- 1 tbsp olive oil
- 1 tbsp lemon juice
- Salt and pepper to taste
- Optional: 1 boiled egg, sliced

Instructions:

1. Place the cooked quinoa as the base layer in the bottom of a bowl.
2. Top the quinoa with arugula or spinach, sliced avocado, smoked salmon, sliced cucumber, and red onion.
3. If using, place the sliced boiled egg in the bowl.
4. Sprinkle capers over the bowl. Drizzle the olive oil and lemon juice over everything. Season with salt and pepper to taste.
5. Serve immediately.

Nutrition Information:

Calories: 550 Protein: 25 g Fat: 40 g Carbohydrates: 27 g Fiber: 9 g Sugar: 5 g

Almond Flour Blueberry Muffins

Prep Time: 15 minutes

Cook Time: 25 minutes

Serving: 12 muffins

Ingredients:

- 2 1/2 cups of almond flour
- 1/2 cup of erythritol (or another sugar substitute)
- 1 tsp baking powder
- 1/4 tsp salt
- 3 large eggs
- 1/3 cup of unsweetened almond milk
- 1/3 cup of coconut oil, melted
- 1 tsp vanilla extract
- 1 cup of fresh or frozen blueberries

Instructions:

1. Preheat the oven to 350°F (175° C). Line a muffin tray with paper liners or spray with nonstick spray.
2. Combine almond flour, erythritol, baking powder, and salt in a large bowl.
3. In a separate bowl, mix the eggs, almond milk, melted coconut oil, and vanilla extract until thoroughly blended.
4. Stir the wet and dry ingredients together until just blended. Gently fold in the blueberries.
5. Spoon the batter into the muffin cups, filling them approximately three-quarters full.
6. Bake for 25 minutes in a preheated oven or until the tops are brown and a toothpick inserted into the middle of each muffin comes out clean.
7. Let the muffins cool in the pan for 5 minutes before transferring to a wire rack to finish cooling.

Nutrition Information:

Calories (per muffin): 220 Protein: 6 g Fat: 18 g Carbohydrates: 9 g Fiber: 3 g Sugar: 4 g

CHAPTER 4: LUNCH RECIPES

Grilled Chicken & Quinoa Salad

Prep Time: 15 minutes

Cook Time: 10 minutes

Serving: 2

Ingredients:

- 2 boneless, skinless chicken breasts
- 1 cup of quinoa, cooked
- 1 avocado, diced
- 1 cup of cherry tomatoes, halved
- 1/2 cucumber, diced
- 1/4 red onion, thinly sliced
- 1/4 cup of feta cheese, crumbled (optional)
- 2 tbsp olive oil
- Juice of 1 lemon
- Salt and pepper to taste
- Optional: fresh herbs like parsley or cilantro, chopped

Instructions:

1. Season the chicken breasts with salt and pepper. Grill 5 minutes per side until thoroughly cooked and the internal temperature reaches 165°F (75°C).
2. Let the chicken rest for a few minutes before slicing thinly.
3. Add cooked quinoa, diced avocado, cherry tomatoes, cucumber, and red onion in a large mixing bowl.
4. Add the grilled chicken pieces to the salad. Drizzle with olive oil and lemon juice. Toss everything to blend, and season with salt and pepper to taste.
5. If desired, garnish with crumbled feta cheese and finely chopped fresh herbs.
6. Serve immediately.

Nutrition Information:

Calories: 500 Protein: 30 g Fat: 28 g Carbohydrates: 35 g Fiber: 8 g Sugar: 5 g

Cauliflower Rice stir-fried with Shrimp

Prep Time: 15 minutes

Cook Time: 10 minutes

Serving: 2

Ingredients:

- 1 pound shrimp, peeled and deveined
- 3 cups of cauliflower rice (from about 1 medium head of cauliflower)
- 1 bell pepper, sliced
- 1 carrot, julienned
- 1/2 onion, sliced
- 2 cloves garlic, minced
- 2 tbsp soy sauce or tamari for a gluten-free option
- 1 tbsp sesame oil
- 1 tsp ginger, grated
- 2 green onions, chopped for garnish
- 1 tbsp olive oil
- Salt and pepper to taste
- Optional: sesame seeds for garnish

Instructions:

1. Heat the olive oil in a large pan or wok over medium-high heat.
2. Sauté the garlic, ginger, and onion for approximately 2 minutes, until aromatic and slightly softened.
3. Increase the heat to high, then add the shrimp to the skillet. Cook for 2-3 minutes or until the shrimp are pink and almost fully cooked.
4. Add the bell pepper and carrot to the skillet. Stir-fry for another 2 minutes, until the veggies are soft but crunchy.
5. Combine the cauliflower rice and soy sauce. Stir everything together and simmer for 3-4 minutes until the cauliflower is soft and everything is well cooked.
6. Drizzle sesame oil over the stir-fry and combine thoroughly.
7. Season with salt and pepper to taste.
8. Serve hot, topped with chopped green onions and sesame seeds if preferred.

Nutrition Information:

Calories: 350 Protein: 35 g Fat: 15 g Carbohydrates: 15 g Fiber: 5 g Sugar: 7 g

Spinach & Avocado Tuna Salad

Prep Time: 10 minutes

Cook Time: 0 minutes

Serving: 2

Ingredients:

- 1 can tuna (in water or olive oil), drained
- 2 cups of fresh spinach, roughly chopped
- 1 ripe avocado, diced
- 1/2 cucumber, diced
- 1/4 red onion, finely chopped
- 1 tbsp lemon juice
- 1 tbsp olive oil
- Salt and pepper to taste
- Optional: 1 tbsp fresh parsley or cilantro, chopped

Instructions:

1. Add the drained tuna, chopped spinach, diced avocado, cucumber, and red onion in a bowl.
2. Drizzle the lemon juice and olive oil over the mixture, tossing gently to incorporate.
3. Season with salt and pepper to taste. If preferred, season with fresh parsley or cilantro.
4. Serve immediately.

Nutrition Information:

Calories: 320 Protein: 25 g Fat: 22 g Carbohydrates: 10 g Fiber: 6 g Sugar: 2 g

Greek Chicken Salad Wrap

Prep Time: 15 minutes

Cook Time: 0 minutes

Serving: 2

Ingredients:

- 1 cup of cooked chicken breast, diced
- 1/2 cup of cucumber, diced
- 1/2 cup of cherry tomatoes, halved
- 1/4 cup of red onion, thinly sliced
- 1/4 cup of Kalamata olives, sliced
- 1/4 cup of feta cheese, crumbled
- 2 tbsp Greek yogurt
- 1 tbsp olive oil
- 1 tbsp lemon juice
- 1/2 tsp dried oregano
- Salt and pepper to taste
- 2 large whole wheat or low-carb wraps
- Optional: Fresh spinach or arugula for added greens

Instructions:

1. Mix the chopped chicken, cucumber, cherry tomatoes, red onion, olives, and feta cheese in a large bowl.
2. In a small bowl, combine the Greek yogurt, olive oil, lemon juice, dried oregano, salt, and pepper.
3. Pour the dressing over the salad and toss to coat.
4. Place the wraps on a clean surface and fill the middle with a handful of spinach or arugula.
5. Divide the Greek chicken salad mixture evenly between the two wraps.
6. Fold the sides of each wrap and roll securely. Serve immediately.

Nutrition Information:

Calories: 400 Protein: 30 g Fat: 20 g Carbohydrates: 30 g Fiber: 6 g Sugar: 5 g

Turkey & Veggie Lettuce Wraps

Prep Time: 10 minutes

Cook Time: 10 minutes

Serving: 2

Ingredients:

- 1 tbsp olive oil
- 1/2 pound ground turkey
- 1 garlic clove, minced
- 1/2 red bell pepper, diced
- 1/2 zucchini, diced
- 1/4 cup of shredded carrots
- 1 tbsp low-sodium soy sauce or tamari for gluten-free
- 1/2 tsp ground ginger
- Salt and pepper to taste
- 6 large lettuce leaves (like butter or romaine lettuce)
- Optional toppings: sliced green onions, sesame seeds, or a drizzle of sriracha

Instructions:

1. Heat the olive oil in a medium-sized pan. Sauté the minced garlic until fragrant, about 1 minute.
2. Add the ground turkey to the skillet. Cook for 5-7 minutes, breaking up with a spoon, until no longer pink.
3. Add the zucchini, bell pepper, and shredded carrots to the skillet. Stir in the veggies and simmer for 3-4 more or until tender.
4. Add the soy sauce and ground ginger, and season with salt and pepper to taste. Cook for a further minute to blend flavors, then remove from heat.
5. Place the turkey and vegetable combination in the center of each lettuce leaf.
6. If preferred, garnish with green onions, sesame seeds, or sriracha. Serve immediately.

Nutrition Information:

Calories: 250 Protein: 25 g Fat: 12 g Carbohydrates: 10 g Fiber: 3 g Sugar: 4 g

Zucchini Noodles with Pesto & Cherry Tomatoes

Prep Time: 10 minutes

Cook Time: 5 minutes

Serving: 2

Ingredients:

- 2 medium zucchinis, spiralized into noodles
- 1 cup of cherry tomatoes, halved
- 1/4 cup of pesto (homemade or store-bought)
- 1 tbsp olive oil
- Salt and pepper to taste
- Optional: grated Parmesan cheese and fresh basil for garnish

Instructions:

1. In a large skillet, heat olive oil over medium heat.
2. Sauté the zucchini noodles in the pan for 2-3 minutes, until they are cooked but still firm.
3. Add the pesto and cherry tomatoes to the skillet. Toss everything together gently, then heat for another 1-2 minutes to soften the tomatoes and coat the noodles with pesto.
4. Season with salt and pepper to taste.
5. Remove from the heat and serve immediately. Garnish with grated Parmesan cheese and fresh basil if preferred.

Nutrition Information:

Calories: 200 Protein: 5 g Fat: 16 g Carbohydrates: 10 g Fiber: 3 g Sugar: 6 g

Steak & Roasted Veggie Bowl

Prep Time: 15 minutes

Cook Time: 25 minutes

Serving: 2

Ingredients:

- 8 oz steak (such as sirloin or flank) seasoned with salt and pepper
- 1 cup of broccoli florets
- 1 cup of cauliflower florets
- 1 red bell pepper, diced
- 1/2 red onion, sliced
- 1 tbsp olive oil
- 1 tsp garlic powder
- 1/2 tsp smoked paprika
- Salt and pepper to taste
- Optional: 1/4 cup of crumbled feta or goat cheese for topping

Instructions:

1. Preheat the oven to 400 °F (200 °C).
2. Combine the broccoli, cauliflower, bell pepper, red onion with olive oil, garlic powder, smoked paprika, salt, and pepper on a baking sheet.
3. Roast the veggies in a preheated oven for 20-25 minutes, turning halfway through or until soft and gently browned.
4. While the veggies roast, preheat a grill pan or skillet over medium-high heat. Cook the steak for 3-4 minutes per side for medium-rare or until desired doneness.
5. Remove the steak from the pan and rest for 5 minutes before slicing thinly.
6. Divide the roasted veggies into two bowl. Top each bowl with sliced steak.
7. If preferred, top with crumbled feta or goat cheese. Serve immediately.

Nutrition Information:

Calories: 450 Protein: 35 g Fat: 25 g Carbohydrates: 18 g Fiber: 6 g Sugar: 6 g

Sesame Salmon Salad

Prep Time: 10 minutes Cook Time: 10 minutes Serving: 2

Ingredients:

- 2 salmon fillets (4 oz each)
- 1 tbsp sesame oil
- 1 tbsp soy sauce or tamari for gluten-free
- 1 tbsp sesame seeds
- 4 cups of mixed salad greens
- 1/2 cucumber, sliced
- 1/2 avocado, sliced
- 1/2 cup of shredded carrots
- 1/4 cup of sliced radishes
- 1 green onion, chopped
- Optional: 1 tbsp chopped fresh cilantro for garnish
- Dressing:
- 2 tbsp rice vinegar
- 1 tbsp olive oil
- 1 tsp sesame oil
- 1 tsp soy sauce or tamari
- 1/2 tsp honey or a low-carb sweetener
- Salt and pepper to taste

Instructions:

1. Cook in a nonstick skillet over medium-high heat. Rub sesame oil and soy sauce into the salmon fillets, then sprinkle with sesame seeds on both sides.
2. Place the salmon in the skillet and cook for 3-4 minutes per side or until desired doneness.
3. While the salmon cooks, prepare the salad by mixing mixed greens, cucumber, avocado, shredded carrots, radishes, and green onion in a large bowl.
4. To make the dressing, combine the rice vinegar, olive oil, sesame oil, soy sauce, honey, salt, and pepper in a small mixing bowl.
5. Once the salmon is cooked, lay it on top of the salad. Drizzle the dressing over the salad and top with cilantro, if desired.
6. Serve immediately.

Nutrition Information:

Calories: 400 Protein: 28 g Fat: 30 g Carbohydrates: 10 g Fiber: 5 g Sugar: 4 g

Cauliflower Crust Veggie Pizza

Prep Time: 20 minutes Cook Time: 25 minutes Serving: 2-3

Ingredients:

- For the crust:
- 1 medium head of cauliflower, grated or riced (about 2 cups)
- 1 large egg
- 1/2 cup of shredded mozzarella cheese
- 1/4 cup of grated Parmesan cheese
- 1/2 tsp Italian seasoning
- Salt and pepper to taste
- For the toppings:
- 1/2 cup of pizza sauce (low-sugar or homemade)
- 1/2 cup of shredded mozzarella cheese
- 1/2 cup of sliced bell peppers (any color)
- 1/4 cup of sliced mushrooms
- 1/4 cup of cherry tomatoes, halved
- 1/4 red onion, thinly sliced
- Optional: fresh basil leaves for garnish

Instructions:

1. Preheat the oven to 400 °F (200 °C). Line a baking sheet with parchment paper.
2. In a microwave-safe bowl, steam the cauliflower rice for 5 minutes or until soft. Allow it to cool somewhat before placing it in a clean kitchen towel and squeezing any excess moisture.
3. Combine the cauliflower rice, egg, mozzarella cheese, parmesan cheese, Italian seasoning, salt, and pepper in a large mixing bowl until a dough forms.
4. Spread the cauliflower mixture on the prepared baking sheet, flattening it into a 1/4-inch-thick circle.
5. Bake for 15 minutes or until the crust is golden and firm.
6. Remove the dough from the oven and sprinkle it with the pizza sauce. Sprinkle with shredded mozzarella, then top with bell peppers, mushrooms, cherry tomatoes, and red onion.
7. Return the pizza to the oven and cook for another 8-10 minutes or until the cheese is melted and bubbling.
8. Garnish with fresh basil leaves, then slice and serve hot.

Nutrition Information:

Calories: 280 (per serving) Protein: 15 g Fat: 16 g Carbohydrates: 14 g Fiber: 4 g Sugar: 5 g

Grilled Halloumi & Arugula Salad

Prep Time: 10 minutes

Cook Time: 5 minutes

Serving: 2

Ingredients:

- 4 oz halloumi cheese, sliced into 1/4-inch thick pieces
- 4 cups of arugula
- 1/2 cup of cherry tomatoes, halved
- 1/2 cucumber, sliced
- 1/4 red onion, thinly sliced
- 1 tbsp olive oil
- Juice of 1/2 lemon
- Salt and pepper to taste
- Optional: 1 tbsp toasted pine nuts for garnish

Instructions:

1. Preheat a nonstick skillet or grill pan to medium-high heat.
2. Add the halloumi slices and heat each side for 1-2 minutes until golden and gently browned. Remove from the pan and put aside.
3. Combine the arugula, cherry tomatoes, cucumber, and red onion in a large mixing bowl.
4. Toss in the olive oil and lemon juice until well coated. Season with salt and pepper to taste.
5. Place the grilled halloumi on top of the salad. Sprinkle with roasted pine nuts if desired.
6. Serve immediately.

Nutrition Information:

Calories: 300 Protein: 15 g Fat: 24 g Carbohydrates: 8 g Fiber: 3 g Sugar: 3 g

Baked Lemon Herb Cod with Spinach

Prep Time: 10 minutes

Cook Time: 15 minutes

Serving: 2

Ingredients:

- 2 cod fillets (about 4 oz each)
- 2 tbsp olive oil
- 1 tbsp fresh lemon juice
- 1 tsp lemon zest
- 1/2 tsp dried thyme
- 1/2 tsp dried parsley
- Salt and pepper to taste
- 2 cups of fresh spinach
- 1 garlic clove, minced
- Optional: lemon slices for garnish

Instructions:

1. Preheat the oven to 400 °F (200 °C). Line a baking sheet with parchment paper or gently coat it with olive oil.
2. In a small mixing bowl, combine the olive oil, lemon juice, zest, thyme, parsley, salt, and pepper.
3. Place the fish fillets on the prepared baking sheet. Brush the lemon herb mixture on the fish, ensuring it's uniformly covered.
4. Bake the fish for 12-15 minutes or until readily flaked with a fork.
5. While the cod is baking, preheat a small skillet over medium. Drizzle with olive oil and chopped garlic. Sauté for 1 minute, until aromatic, and then add the spinach. Cook, tossing regularly, until wilted, approximately 2-3 minutes.
6. Serve the cod fillets on a bed of sautéed spinach, topped with lemon slices if preferred.

Nutrition Information:

Calories: 250 Protein: 28 g Fat: 14 g Carbohydrates: 4 g Fiber: 1 g Sugar: 0 g

Quinoa & Roasted Veggie Buddha Bowl

Prep Time: 15 minutes Cook Time: 25 minutes Serving: 2

Ingredients:

- 1/2 cup of quinoa, rinsed
- 1 cup of water or vegetable broth
- 1 cup of sweet potato, diced
- 1 cup of broccoli florets
- 1/2 red bell pepper, sliced
- 1/2 zucchini, sliced
- 2 tbsp olive oil
- Salt and pepper to taste
- 1/2 tsp paprika
- 1/2 tsp garlic powder
- 1 cup of fresh spinach
- 1/2 avocado, sliced
- For the dressing:
- 2 tbsp tahini
- 1 tbsp lemon juice
- 1 tbsp water (or more to thin, if needed)
- Salt and pepper to taste
- Optional: a pinch of cayenne for a hint of spice

Instructions:

1. Preheat the oven to 400 °F (200 °C). Line a baking sheet with parchment paper.
2. Mix the quinoa and water (or veggie broth) in a small saucepan. Bring to a boil, then decrease heat, cover, and simmer for approximately 15 minutes or until the quinoa is cooked and the water has been absorbed. Fluff with a fork, then set aside.
3. While the quinoa cooks, combine the sweet potato, broccoli, red bell pepper, and zucchini with olive oil, salt, pepper, paprika, and garlic powder. Spread the veggies equally on the prepared baking sheet.
4. Roast the veggies for 20-25 minutes, tossing halfway, until soft and lightly browned.
5. In a small mixing bowl, combine the tahini, lemon juice, water, salt, and pepper to make the dressing. Add more water if necessary to get the desired consistency.
6. To make the bowls, split the cooked quinoa into two bowls. Add the roasted vegetables, spinach, and avocado to the quinoa.
7. Drizzle with tahini dressing and serve immediately.

Nutrition Information:

Calories: 450 Protein: 12 g Fat: 24 g Carbohydrates: 50 g Fiber: 12 g Sugar: 6 g

Thai Chicken Lettuce Cup

Prep Time: 10 minutes Cook Time: 10 minutes Serving: 2

Ingredients:

- 1 tbsp olive oil
- 1/2 pound ground chicken
- 2 cloves garlic, minced
- 1/2 red bell pepper, diced
- 1/4 cup of shredded carrots
- 2 green onions, chopped
- 1 tbsp soy sauce or tamari for gluten-free
- 1 tbsp fish sauce
- 1 tbsp lime juice
- 1/2 tsp honey or a low-carb sweetener
- 1/4 tsp chili flakes
- Salt and pepper to taste
- 6-8 large lettuce leaves
- Optional toppings: chopped fresh cilantro, chopped peanuts, and lime wedges

Instructions:

1. In a pan, heat olive oil over medium-high heat. Add the minced garlic and simmer for about 1 minute or until fragrant.
2. Add the ground chicken to the skillet and cook, breaking it up with a spoon, until no longer pink (approximately 5-7 minutes).
3. Add the diced red bell pepper, shredded carrots, and green onions to the skillet. Stir and simmer for 2-3 minutes until the veggies are soft.
4. Combine the soy sauce, fish sauce, lime juice, honey, and chili flakes in a small mixing bowl. Pour the sauce over the chicken and vegetable mixture, tossing thoroughly to incorporate. Cook for 1-2 minutes more or until the flavors mix.
5. Season with salt and pepper to taste, then remove from the heat.
6. Place the chicken mixture in the center of each lettuce leaf. Optional garnishes include chopped cilantro, peanuts, and a splash of lime juice.
7. Serve immediately.

Nutrition Information:

Calories: 280 Protein: 25 g Fat: 15 g Carbohydrates: 10 g Fiber: 3 g Sugar: 3 g

Chicken Caesar Salad with Kale

Prep Time: 15 minutes

Cook Time: 10 minutes

Servings: 2

Ingredients:

- 2 cups of kale, stems removed, chopped
- 1 cup of romaine lettuce, chopped
- 1 grilled chicken breast, sliced
- 2 tbsp grated Parmesan cheese
- 2 tbsp Greek yogurt
- 1 tbsp olive oil
- 1 tbsp lemon juice
- 1 tsp Dijon mustard
- 1 garlic clove, minced
- Salt and pepper to taste
- Optional: a few whole grain croutons for added crunch

Instructions:

1. In a large mixing bowl, mix the kale and romaine lettuce.
2. Place the sliced grilled chicken breast on top.
3. In a separate small bowl, combine Greek yogurt, olive oil, lemon juice, Dijon mustard, chopped garlic, salt, and pepper.
4. Pour the dressing over the salad and toss to coat evenly. If preferred, top with Parmesan cheese and croutons.
5. Serve immediately.

Nutrition (per serving):

Calories: 280 Protein: 30g Carbohydrates: 8g Fiber: 3g Fat: 14g

Blackened Shrimp & Cauliflower Grits

Prep Time: 15 minutes Cook Time: 20 minutes Servings: 2

Ingredients

- For the Shrimp:
- 1/2 lb large shrimp, peeled and deveined
- 1 tbsp olive oil
- 1/2 tsp paprika
- 1/2 tsp garlic powder
- 1/2 tsp onion powder
- 1/4 tsp cayenne pepper (optional for heat)
- Salt and black pepper, to taste
- Fresh parsley, chopped, for garnish
- For the Cauliflower Grits:
- 1 medium head of cauliflower, chopped into florets
- 1/4 cup of unsweetened almond milk (or any milk alternative)
- 1 tbsp nutritional yeast (for a cheesy flavor)
- 1/2 tsp garlic powder
- Salt and black pepper, to taste

Instructions

1. Bring a saucepan of water to a boil. Add the cauliflower florets. Boil for 8–10 minutes or until very tender. Drain the cauliflower and add it to a food processor or blender.
2. Add the almond milk, nutritional yeast, garlic powder, salt, and pepper to the cauliflower. Blend until smooth and creamy, adding more almond milk as needed. Set aside to stay warm.
3. Mix the paprika, garlic powder, onion powder, cayenne pepper (if using), salt, and black pepper in a bowl.
4. Pat the shrimp dry, then toss with olive oil and the spice mixture to coat evenly.
5. Cook in a skillet over medium-high heat. Once heated, add the shrimp and cook for 2-3 minutes on each side or until opaque and fully cooked. Remove from heat.
6. Divide the cauliflower grits across two bowls and top with the blackened shrimp.
7. Garnish with chopped parsley and serve immediately.

Nutrition Information (per serving)

Calories: 230 Protein: 22g Carbohydrates: 10g Fiber: 4g Total Fat: 10g Sodium: 680mg

Mediterranean Veggie Bowl with Hummus

Prep Time: 15 minutes Cook Time: 10 minutes Servings: 2

Ingredients

- 1 cup of cooked quinoa
- 1/2 cup of cherry tomatoes, halved
- 1/2 cucumber, diced
- 1/2 red bell pepper, diced
- 1/4 cup of Kalamata olives, sliced
- 1/4 cup of red onion, thinly sliced
- 1/4 cup of crumbled feta cheese (optional)
- 1/2 avocado, sliced
- 1/2 cup of canned chickpeas, drained and rinsed
- 1 tbsp tahini
- 1 tbsp lemon juice
- 1 clove garlic, minced
- 1/4 tsp cumin
- 2-3 tbsp water (adjust for consistency)
- Salt and pepper, to taste
- 1 tbsp extra-virgin olive oil
- 1 tbsp lemon juice
- Salt and pepper, to taste
- Fresh parsley, chopped, for garnish

Instructions

1. Mix chickpeas, tahini, lemon juice, garlic, cumin, salt, and pepper in a food processor. Blend until smooth, then add water and a spoonful until you achieve the appropriate consistency. Set aside.
2. To make the dressing, combine the olive oil, lemon juice, salt, and pepper in a small mixing bowl.
3. Divide the cooked quinoa into two bowls. Place the cherry tomatoes, cucumber, bell pepper, olives, red onion, feta (if using), and avocado around the quinoa.
4. Place a heaping dollop of hummus in each bowl.
5. Drizzle the dressing on the vegetables and quinoa. Garnish with chopped parsley and serve immediately.

Nutrition Information (per serving)

Calories: 420 Protein: 14g Carbohydrates: 42g Fiber: 10g Total Fat: 22g

Low-Carb Turkey Avocado Wrap

Prep Time: 10 minutes

Cook Time: 5 minutes

Servings: 2

Ingredients

- 4 large lettuce leaves
- 6 oz turkey breast slices
- 1/2 avocado, sliced
- 1/4 cup of shredded cheddar cheese (optional)
- 2 tbsp hummus or mustard
- 1/4 cup of cucumber, thinly sliced
- 1/4 cup of tomato, thinly sliced
- Salt and pepper, to taste
- Fresh parsley, chopped, for garnish (optional)

Instructions

1. Place the lettuce leaves flat on a clean surface, ensuring they are large enough to wrap around the filling.
2. Spread 1 spoonful of hummus or mustard over each lettuce leaf.
3. Layer the turkey slices on the lettuce, then add avocado, cucumber, and tomato.
4. Season with salt and pepper to taste and sprinkle with shredded cheddar cheese (if using).
5. To make a wrap, carefully fold the edges of the lettuce leaves and roll securely.
6. Cut the wraps in half and decorate with fresh parsley, if desired. Serve immediately.

Nutrition Information (per serving)

Calories: 270 Protein: 25g Carbohydrates: 7g Fiber: 5g Total Fat: 17g Sodium: 780mg

Asian Ginger Chicken & Cabbage Slaw

Prep Time: 15 minutes

Cook Time: 20 minutes

Servings: 2

Ingredients

- 2 boneless, skinless chicken breasts
- 1 tbsp olive oil
- 2 tbsp fresh ginger, minced
- 2 cloves garlic, minced
- 2 tbsp soy sauce
- 1 tbsp rice vinegar
- 1 tbsp honey (optional for sweetness)
- 1/2 tsp sesame oil
- Salt and pepper, to taste
- 2 cups of shredded green cabbage
- 1 cup of shredded purple cabbage
- 1/2 cup of shredded carrots
- 1/4 cup of green onions, thinly sliced
- 1/4 cup of cilantro, chopped
- 1 tbsp sesame seeds (optional)
- 2 tbsp soy sauce (or coconut aminos)
- 1 tbsp rice vinegar
- 1 tbsp fresh lime juice
- 1 tsp sesame oil
- 1 tsp honey or maple syrup
- 1/4 tsp red pepper flakes (optional for heat)
- Salt and pepper, to taste

Instructions

1. In a medium-sized pan, heat the olive oil. Season the chicken breasts with salt and pepper.
2. Cook the chicken in the skillet for 6-7 minutes per side or until well-cooked and golden brown. Remove the chicken from the skillet and put it aside.
3. In the same pan, combine the minced ginger and garlic. Sauté for 1–2 minutes or until aromatic.

4. Combine the soy sauce, rice vinegar, honey (if using), and sesame oil. Allow the sauce to boil for 2-3 minutes until slightly thickened.
5. When the chicken is done, slice it into thin strips and return it to the skillet, stirring it with the ginger sauce until covered.
6. Add green cabbage, purple cabbage, shredded carrots, green onions, and cilantro in a large bowl. Toss to combine thoroughly.
7. In a small mixing bowl, combine the soy sauce, rice vinegar, lime juice, sesame oil, honey, red pepper flakes (if desired), salt, and pepper.
8. Toss the cabbage slaw in the dressing until well coated. Serve the ginger chicken over the cabbage slaw, topped with sesame seeds if desired.

Nutrition Information (per serving)

Calories: 350 Protein: 40g Carbohydrates: 18g Fiber: 6g Total Fat: 16g

Lemon Garlic Zoodles with Shredded Chicken

Prep Time: 15 minutes Cook Time: 15 minutes Servings: 2

Ingredients:

- 2 medium zucchini, spiralized (zoodles)
- 1 tbsp olive oil
- 2 cloves garlic, minced
- 1 lemon, juiced and zested
- 1 cup of cooked, shredded chicken breast
- 1/4 tsp sea salt
- 1/4 tsp black pepper
- 1/4 tsp red pepper flakes (optional)
- 2 tbsp fresh parsley, chopped
- 1/4 cup of grated Parmesan cheese
- Lemon wedges (for serving)

Instructions:

1. Use a spiralizer or julienne peeler to make zoodles from the zucchini. Set aside.
2. In a large skillet, heat olive oil over medium heat. Sauté minced garlic for about 1 minute, until aromatic.
3. Toss the shredded chicken in the pan with the garlic until well coated. Cook for 2-3 minutes, until well heated.

4. Add the zoodles to the skillet. Sauté the zoodles for about 2-3 minutes, turning regularly, until soft yet slightly crunchy.
5. Squeeze lemon juice over the zoodles and sprinkle with lemon zest. Season with salt, pepper, and red pepper flakes (if desired).
6. Toss everything together and heat for another minute to let the flavors combine. Remove from the heat and season with fresh parsley and grated Parmesan (if using).
7. Serve immediately, with lemon slices to the side.

Nutrition Information (Per Serving):

Calories: 280 Protein: 30g Carbohydrates: 10g Dietary Fiber: 3g Sugar: 5g Fat: 12g

Low-Carb Taco Salad

Prep Time: 15 minutes

Cook Time: 10 minutes

Servings: 4

Ingredients:

- 1 pound ground beef (lean)
- 1 tbsp olive oil
- 1 medium onion, diced
- 2 cloves garlic, minced
- 1 tbsp chili powder
- 1 tsp cumin
- 1/2 tsp paprika
- 1/2 tsp sea salt
- 1/4 tsp black pepper
- 4 cups of romaine lettuce, chopped
- 1 cup of cherry tomatoes, halved
- 1/2 cup of cucumber, diced
- 1/4 cup of red onion, thinly sliced
- 1/2 cup of shredded cheddar cheese (optional)
- 1 avocado, sliced
- 1/4 cup of fresh cilantro, chopped
- Juice of 1 lime

Instructions:

1. In a large skillet, heat olive oil over medium heat. Sauté the diced onion for 3-4 minutes, until softened.
2. Add the minced garlic and heat for 30 seconds or until fragrant.
3. Add the ground meat to the skillet. Cook, breaking it up with a spatula, until browned, approximately 5-7 minutes.
4. Season the meat with chili powder, cumin, paprika, salt, and pepper. Stir well to mix. Cook for another 2-3 minutes until the spices are well integrated. Remove from the heat and put aside.
5. Mix the romaine lettuce, cherry tomatoes, cucumber, and red onion in a large salad bowl.
6. Sprinkle the salad with seasoned ground beef, shredded cheddar cheese (if using), avocado slices, and cilantro.
7. Squeeze fresh lime juice over the salad and gently toss to combine.
8. Serve immediately.

Nutrition Information (Per Serving):

Calories: 320 Protein: 25g Carbohydrates: 8g Dietary Fiber: 4g Sugar: 3g Fat: 22g

CHAPTER 5: DINNER RECIPES

Baked Salmon with Asparagus

Prep Time: 10 minutes Cook Time: 20 minutes Servings: 4

Ingredients:

- Four salmon fillets (about 6 oz each)
- 1 pound asparagus, trimmed
- 2 tbsp olive oil
- 2 cloves garlic, minced
- 1 lemon, thinly sliced
- 1 lemon, juiced
- 1 tsp sea salt
- 1/2 tsp black pepper
- 1 tsp dried oregano
- 1 tsp smoked paprika
- Fresh parsley, chopped (for garnish)

Instructions:

1. Preheat the oven to 400 °F (200 °C). Line a baking sheet with parchment or aluminum foil.
2. Arrange the salmon fillets in the middle of the baking sheet. Arrange the asparagus around the fish.
3. Drizzle olive oil on the fish and asparagus. Season with minced garlic. Season the salmon with salt and pepper, oregano, and smoky paprika.
4. Arrange the lemon slices on top of the salmon fillets, then squeeze the juice of one lemon equally across the entire sheet.
5. Bake for 15-20 minutes in a preheated oven until the salmon is cooked and easily flaked with a fork and the asparagus is soft.
6. Remove from the oven and sprinkle with fresh parsley to serve.
7. Serve immediately, with more lemon wedges if preferred.

Nutrition Information (Per Serving):

Calories: 350 Protein: 30g Carbohydrates: 5g Dietary Fiber: 2g Sugar: 2g Fat: 22g

Garlic & Herb Roasted Chicken with Brussels Sprouts

Prep Time: 15 minutes Cook Time: 45 minutes Servings: 4

Ingredients:

- 4 bone-in, skin-on chicken thighs
- 1 pound Brussels sprouts, trimmed and halved
- 3 tbsp olive oil
- 4 cloves garlic, minced
- 1 tbsp fresh rosemary, chopped
- 1 tbsp fresh thyme, chopped
- 1 tsp dried oregano
- 1 tsp sea salt
- 1/2 tsp black pepper
- 1 lemon, juiced
- Zest of 1 lemon
- 1/4 cup of chicken broth
- Fresh parsley, chopped (for garnish)

Instructions:

1. Preheat the oven to 400 °F (200 °C). Line a large baking sheet with parchment paper or gently oil it.
2. Combine the Brussels sprouts, 1 tbsp olive oil, salt, and pepper in a large bowl. Spread them equally on one half of the baking sheet.
3. Pat the chicken thighs dry with paper towels. Rub them in the remaining 2 tbsp olive oil, ensuring they're equally covered.
4. Combine the minced garlic, rosemary, thyme, oregano, lemon zest, salt, and pepper in a small bowl.
5. Rub the garlic and herb mixture evenly on the chicken thighs, pushing it into the skin.
6. Arrange the seasoned chicken thighs on a baking sheet alongside the Brussels sprouts.
7. Drizzle the lemon juice and broth over the chicken and Brussels sprouts.
8. Roast in an oven for 40-45 minutes until the chicken skin is brown and crispy and the internal temperature reaches 165°F (74°C).
9. Remove from the oven and allow to cool for 5 minutes. Sprinkle with fresh parsley before serving.

Nutrition Information (Per Serving):

Calories: 410 Protein: 28g Carbohydrates: 10g Dietary Fiber: 4g Sugar: 2g Fat: 28g

Zucchini Lasagna with Ground Turkey

Prep Time: 20 minutes Cook Time: 40 minutes Servings: 6

Ingredients:

- 2 large zucchini, sliced lengthwise into thin strips
- 1 pound ground turkey
- 1 tbsp olive oil
- 1 medium onion, diced
- 3 cloves garlic, minced
- 1 can (14 oz) crushed tomatoes
- 1/2 cup of tomato sauce (low-sugar)
- 1 tsp dried basil
- 1 tsp dried oregano
- 1/2 tsp sea salt
- 1/4 tsp black pepper
- 1 cup of ricotta cheese (or cottage cheese for a lower-fat option)
- 1 large egg
- 1/2 cup of shredded mozzarella cheese (optional)
- 1/4 cup of grated Parmesan cheese
- Fresh basil leaves (for garnish)

Instructions:

1. Preheat the oven to 375° Fahrenheit (190° Celsius). Lightly butter a 9x13-inch baking dish.
2. Use a mandolin or a sharp knife to slice the zucchini into thin, uniform strips. Lay the strips on a paper towel, sprinkle with salt, and let them rest for 10 minutes to remove excess moisture. Before usage, be sure to pat it dry.
3. In a large skillet, heat olive oil over medium heat. Sauté the diced onion for 3-4 minutes, until softened. Add the minced garlic and cook for a further 30 seconds.
4. Add the ground turkey to the skillet. Cook, breaking it up with a spatula, until browned, approximately 5-7 minutes.
5. Combine the crushed tomatoes, tomato sauce, basil, oregano, salt, and pepper. Reduce the heat and simmer for 10 minutes, allowing the flavors to combine.
6. In a small bowl, mix the ricotta cheese and egg. Mix until smooth.

7. Spread a thin layer of turkey sauce on the bottom of the baking dish. Layer the zucchini slices first, followed by the ricotta mixture. Repeat the layers, finishing with turkey sauce on top.
8. Sprinkle the top with mozzarella and Parmesan cheese (if using).
9. Cover with aluminum foil and bake for 20 minutes. Remove the cover and bake for 15-20 minutes or until the cheese is bubbling and golden brown.
10. Allow the lasagna to rest for ten minutes before slicing. Garnish with fresh basil leaves.

Nutrition Information (Per Serving):

Calories: 280 Protein: 25g Carbohydrates: 8g Dietary Fiber: 2g Sugar: 5g Fat: 15g

Cauliflower Crust Margherita Pizza

Prep Time: 20 minutes

Cook Time: 30 minutes

Servings: 4

Ingredients:

- For the Cauliflower Crust:
- 1 medium head of cauliflower, riced (about 4 cups)
- 1/2 cup of shredded mozzarella cheese
- 1/4 cup of grated Parmesan cheese
- 1 large egg
- 1 tsp dried oregano
- 1/2 tsp garlic powder
- 1/2 tsp sea salt
- For the Toppings:
- 1/2 cup of tomato sauce (no added sugar)
- 1 cup of fresh mozzarella cheese, sliced
- 1/2 cup of cherry tomatoes, halved
- 1/4 cup of fresh basil leaves
- 1 tsp olive oil
- Pinch of sea salt
- Freshly ground black pepper (to taste)

Instructions:

1. Preheat the oven to 425° Fahrenheit (220° Celsius). Cover a baking sheet or pizza stone with parchment paper.
2. Place the cauliflower rice in a microwave-safe bowl and cook for 4-5 minutes until softened. Allow it to cool slightly.
3. Place the cooked cauliflower rice on a clean kitchen towel. Wrap firmly and push out as much liquid as possible for a crispy crust.
4. Combine the cauliflower, mozzarella, Parmesan, egg, oregano, garlic powder, and salt in a large mixing bowl. Mix well until dough forms.
5. Spread the cauliflower mixture on the baking sheet and flatten it into a thin, even circle (approximately 1/4 inch thick).
6. Bake the crust in a preheated oven for 15-20 minutes, until golden brown and firm.
7. Remove the crust from the oven and spread it with a thin layer of tomato sauce. Top with slices of fresh mozzarella, cherry tomatoes, and basil leaves.
8. Drizzle with olive oil, then season with sea salt and black pepper.
9. Return the pizza to the oven and cook for another 10-12 minutes or until the cheese is melted and bubbling.
10. Remove from the oven and allow it to cool for a few minutes. Slice and serve hot, garnishing with more basil leaves if preferred.

Nutrition Information (Per Serving):

Calories: 210 Protein: 12g Carbohydrates: 8g Dietary Fiber: 3g Sugar: 4g Fat: 14g

Keto-Friendly Stuffed Bell Peppers

Prep Time: 15 minutes Cook Time: 30 minutes Servings: 4

Ingredients:

- 4 large bell peppers halved and seeds removed
- 1 tbsp olive oil
- 1 pound ground beef (or ground turkey)
- 1 small onion, diced
- 2 cloves garlic, minced
- 1 can (14 oz) diced tomatoes, drained
- 1/2 cup of cauliflower rice
- 1 tsp dried oregano
- 1 tsp smoked paprika
- 1/2 tsp sea salt
- 1/4 tsp black pepper
- 1 cup of shredded cheddar cheese (or mozzarella)
- Fresh parsley, chopped (for garnish)

Instructions:

1. Preheat the oven to 375° Fahrenheit (190° Celsius). Lightly butter a baking dish. Place the bell pepper halves in the bowl, cut side up.
2. In a large skillet, heat olive oil over medium heat. Sauté the diced onion for 3-4 minutes, until softened. Add the minced garlic and cook for a further 30 seconds.
3. Add the ground beef to the skillet and cook, breaking it up with a spatula, until browned, about 5-7 minutes. Drain any extra fat.
4. Combine the chopped tomatoes, cauliflower rice, oregano, smoked paprika, salt, and pepper. Cook for 5-7 minutes or until the mixture is thoroughly blended and cooked.
5. Spoon the meat and cauliflower mixture equally into each bell pepper half, gently pushing to fill.
6. Top each filled pepper with a liberal amount of shredded cheese.
7. Cover the baking dish with aluminum foil and bake for 20 minutes. Remove the cover and bake for 10 minutes or until the cheese is melted and bubbling.
8. Garnish with fresh parsley before serving.

Nutrition Information (Per Serving):

Calories: 320 Protein: 25g Carbohydrates: 10g Dietary Fiber: 3g Sugar: 5g

Beef & Broccoli Stir-Fry

Prep Time: 15 minutes Cook Time: 15 minutes Servings: 4

Ingredients:

- 1 pound beef sirloin, thinly sliced
- 3 cups of broccoli florets
- 2 tbsp olive oil (or avocado oil), divided
- 3 cloves garlic, minced
- 1/4 cup of low-sodium soy sauce
- 2 tbsp beef broth
- 1 tbsp rice vinegar
- 1 tbsp sesame oil
- 1 tsp ground ginger
- 1/4 tsp red pepper flakes (optional)
- 1 tsp sesame seeds (for garnish)
- 2 green onions, sliced (for garnish)

Instructions:

1. Pat the meat slices dry with a paper towel. This helps to produce a nice sear. Set aside.
2. In a small mixing bowl, combine the soy sauce, beef broth, rice vinegar, sesame oil, ground ginger, and red pepper flakes (if using). Set the sauce mixture aside.
3. Heat 1 tbsp olive oil in a large pan or wok over medium-high heat. Sauté the broccoli florets until they are green and tender-crisp, about 3 to 4 minutes. Place the broccoli on a platter and put aside.
4. In the same skillet, heat the last tbsp of olive oil. Add the sliced meat and cook for 2-3 minutes per side until browned.
5. Cook the minced garlic in the pan for 30 seconds or until fragrant.
6. Pour the prepared sauce mixture into the skillet, stirring to coat the meat evenly. Bring to a boil and cook for 2-3 minutes, until the sauce thickens slightly.
7. Return the broccoli to the skillet and toss until evenly coated with sauce and cooked.
8. Remove from the heat and garnish with sesame seeds and chopped green onions.
9. Serve hot with cauliflower rice for a low-carb dinner.

Nutrition Information (Per Serving):

Calories: 280 Protein: 24g Carbohydrates: 10g Dietary Fiber: 3g Sugar: 2g Fat: 15g

Spaghetti Squash Bolognese

Prep Time: 15 minutes Cook Time: 45 minutes Servings: 4

Ingredients:

- 1 large spaghetti squash
- 1 tbsp olive oil
- 1 pound ground beef
- 1 small onion, diced
- 3 cloves garlic, minced
- 1 can (14 oz) crushed tomatoes
- 1/2 cup of tomato sauce (no sugar added)
- 1/2 cup of beef broth
- 1 tsp dried oregano
- 1 tsp dried basil
- 1/2 tsp sea salt
- 1/4 tsp black pepper
- 1/4 tsp red pepper flakes (optional)
- Fresh parsley, chopped (for garnish)
- Grated Parmesan cheese (optional for serving)

Instructions:

1. Preheat the oven to 400 °F (200 °C). Line a baking sheet with parchment paper.
2. Cut the spaghetti squash in half lengthwise, then scrape out the seeds. Drizzle some olive oil inside and season with salt and pepper. Place the squash halves, cut side down, on the baking sheet.
3. Roast the squash for 35-40 minutes or until the flesh is soft and easy to scrape with a fork. Allow it to cool slightly before scraping away the spaghetti-like threads. Set aside.
4. While the squash is roasting, warm the olive oil in a large pan over medium heat. Sauté the diced onion for 3-4 minutes, until softened. Add the minced garlic and cook for a further 30 seconds.
5. Add the ground meat to the skillet. Cook, breaking it up with a spatula, until browned, approximately 7-8 minutes. Drain any extra fat.
6. Add the crushed tomatoes, tomato sauce, beef broth, oregano, basil, salt, black pepper, and red pepper flakes (if desired). Bring the sauce to a boil and cook for 15-20 minutes, stirring regularly, until thick.
7. Divide the roasted spaghetti squash into serving bowls. Top with the Bolognese sauce.
8. Garnish with fresh parsley and grated Parmesan cheese (optional).

Nutrition Information (Per Serving):

Calories: 310 Protein: 22g Carbohydrates: 14g Dietary Fiber: 5g Sugar: 7g Fat: 18g

Seared Scallops with Zoodles

Prep Time: 10 minutes Cook Time: 10 minutes Servings: 2

Ingredients:

- 12 large sea scallops, patted dry
- 2 medium zucchini, spiralized
- 2 tbsp olive oil (divided)
- 2 cloves garlic, minced
- 1 lemon, juiced and zested
- 1/4 tsp sea salt
- 1/4 tsp black pepper
- 1/4 tsp red pepper flakes (optional)
- 2 tbsp fresh parsley, chopped (for garnish)
- Lemon wedges (for serving)

Instructions:

1. Pat the scallops dry with paper towels. Season each side with salt and pepper.
2. Heat 1 tbsp olive oil in a large pan over medium-high heat. Once heated, add the scallops in a single layer, taking care not to overcrowd the pan.
3. Sear the scallops on each side for 2-3 minutes until a golden brown crust develops. Remove the scallops from the skillet and put them aside.
4. In the same skillet, combine the remaining olive oil and minced garlic. Sauté for approximately 30 seconds until aromatic.
5. Add the zoodles to the skillet and cook for 2-3 minutes, stirring regularly, until cooked but slightly crunchy.
6. Squeeze lemon juice over the zoodles and sprinkle with lemon zest. Sprinkle with salt, pepper, and red pepper flakes (if using).
7. Return the scallops to the skillet and warm quickly, spooning the lemon garlic sauce.
8. Serve immediately, topped with fresh parsley and lemon slices on the side.

Nutrition Information (Per Serving):

Calories: 280 Protein: 25g Carbohydrates: 8g Dietary Fiber: 3g Sugar: 5g Fat: 16g

Grilled Shrimp with Cilantro Lime Cauliflower Rice

Prep Time: 15 minutes

Cook Time: 15 minutes

Servings: 4

Ingredients:

- 1 pound large shrimp, peeled and deveined
- 2 tbsp olive oil
- 2 cloves garlic, minced
- Juice of 1 lime
- 1 tsp smoked paprika
- 1/2 tsp ground cumin
- 1/2 tsp sea salt
- 1/4 tsp black pepper
- 1/4 tsp red pepper flakes (optional)
- 1 medium head of cauliflower, riced (about 4 cups)
- 1 tbsp olive oil
- 2 cloves garlic, minced
- Juice of 1 lime
- Zest of 1 lime
- 1/4 cup of fresh cilantro, chopped
- 1/2 tsp sea salt
- 1/4 tsp black pepper

Instructions:

1. Mix the shrimp, olive oil, minced garlic, lime juice, smoked paprika, cumin, salt, pepper, and red pepper flakes (if using). Toss to coat evenly. Allow it to marinade for 10-15 minutes.
2. Heat 1 tbsp olive oil in a large pan over medium heat. Sauté the minced garlic for 30 seconds, until aromatic.
3. Cook the cauliflower rice in the pan for 5-7 minutes, turning often, until cooked.
4. Combine the lime juice, zest, cilantro, salt, and pepper. Mix well and heat for 1-2 minutes more. Remove from the heat and set aside.
5. Preheat a grill pan or outdoor grill to medium-high heat. Grill the shrimp for 2-3 minutes per side until pink and opaque.

6. Divide the cilantro lime cauliflower rice among plates. Top with the grilled shrimp and garnish with more cilantro and lime wedges.

Nutrition Information (Per Serving):

Calories: 220 Protein: 22g Carbohydrates: 8g Dietary Fiber: 3g Sugar: 3g Fat: 12g

Low-Carb Turkey Meatloaf

Prep Time: 15 minutes Cook Time: 50 minutes Servings: 6

Ingredients:

- 1 1/2 pounds ground turkey
- 1/2 cup of almond flour
- 1 small onion, finely diced
- 2 cloves garlic, minced
- 1 large egg
- 1/4 cup of unsweetened ketchup (low-sugar)
- 2 tbsp fresh parsley, chopped
- 1 tbsp Worcestershire sauce
- 1 tsp dried oregano
- 1 tsp smoked paprika
- 1/2 tsp sea salt
- 1/2 tsp black pepper
- For the Glaze:
- 1/4 cup of unsweetened ketchup
- 1 tbsp Dijon mustard
- 1 tbsp apple cider vinegar

Instructions:

1. Preheat the oven to 375° Fahrenheit (190° Celsius). Line a baking sheet with parchment paper, or gently butter a loaf pan.
2. Add ground turkey, almond flour, chopped onion, minced garlic, egg, ketchup, parsley, Worcestershire sauce, oregano, smoky paprika, salt, and pepper in a large mixing bowl. Mix thoroughly until all of the ingredients are equally combined.
3. Form the mixture into a loaf and lay it on the prepared baking sheet.
4. Combine the ketchup, Dijon mustard, and apple cider vinegar in a small bowl. Apply the glaze evenly on the top of the meatloaf.

5. Bake for 45-50 minutes until the internal temperature reaches 165°F (74°C). Allow the meatloaf to rest for 5–10 minutes before slicing.
6. If preferred, slice and garnish with more fresh parsley.

Nutrition Information (Per Serving):

Calories: 230 Protein: 24g Carbohydrates: 5g Dietary Fiber: 2g Sugar: 2g Fat: 12g

Moroccan-Spiced Chicken with Spinach

Prep Time: 10 minutes

Cook Time: 25 minutes

Servings: 4

Ingredients:

- 1 1/2 pounds boneless, skinless chicken thighs
- 2 tbsp olive oil, divided
- 1 tsp ground cumin
- 1 tsp ground coriander
- 1 tsp ground paprika
- 1/2 tsp ground cinnamon
- 1/4 tsp cayenne pepper (optional)
- 1/2 tsp sea salt
- 1/4 tsp black pepper
- 1 medium onion, thinly sliced
- 3 cloves garlic, minced
- 1/2 cup of chicken broth
- 1/4 cup of fresh lemon juice
- 6 cups of fresh baby spinach
- 1/4 cup of chopped fresh cilantro (for garnish)
- Lemon wedges (for serving)

Instructions:

1. Combine cumin, coriander, paprika, cinnamon, cayenne pepper, salt, and black pepper in a small bowl. Rub the spice mixture equally on both sides of the chicken thighs.

2. Heat 1 tbsp olive oil in a large pan over medium-high heat. Cook the chicken thighs for 4-5 minutes per side until browned. Remove the chicken from the skillet and put it aside.
3. In the same skillet, heat the remaining tbsp olive oil. Sauté the sliced onion for 3-4 minutes, until softened. Add the minced garlic and heat for another 30 seconds or until fragrant.
4. Pour in the chicken stock and lemon juice, scraping out any browned pieces at the bottom of the skillet. Heat the mixture to a simmer.
5. Return the chicken thighs to the skillet. Cover and heat for 10 to 12 minutes or until the chicken is well cooked.
6. Stir in the spinach and cook for approximately 2-3 minutes or until it has wilted.
7. Transfer the chicken and spinach to bowl. Sprinkle with chopped cilantro and serve with lemon wedges on the side.

Nutrition Information (Per Serving):

Calories: 280 Protein: 28g Carbohydrates: 7g Dietary Fiber: 3g Sugar: 2g Fat: 15g

Slow-Cooked Beef Stew with Veggies

Prep Time: 20 minutes Cook Time: 6-8 hours (low) or 4-5 hours (high) Servings: 6

Ingredients:

- 2 pounds beef stew meat, cut into 1-inch cubes
- 2 tbsp olive oil
- 1 medium onion, diced
- 3 cloves garlic, minced
- 4 cups of beef broth (low-sodium)
- 1 can (14 oz) diced tomatoes (no added sugar)
- 2 tbsp tomato paste
- 2 medium carrots, sliced
- 2 stalks celery, sliced
- 2 cups of cauliflower florets
- 1 cup of turnips, peeled and diced (low-carb potato substitute)
- 1 tsp dried thyme
- 1 tsp dried rosemary
- 1 bay leaf
- 1/2 tsp smoked paprika
- 1/2 tsp sea salt

- 1/4 tsp black pepper
- 1/4 cup of fresh parsley, chopped (for garnish)

Instructions:

1. Heat olive oil in a large pan over medium-high heat. Add the meat cubes and brown on all sides (5-7 minutes). Transfer the meat to a slow cooker.
2. In the same skillet, combine the chopped onion and garlic. Sauté for 2-3 minutes, until aromatic, before transferring to the slow cooker.
3. Combine the beef broth, diced tomatoes, and tomato paste in the slow cooker and stir well to mix.
4. Combine the carrots, celery, cauliflower florets, and turnips in the slow cooker.
5. Sprinkle with thyme, rosemary, smoked paprika, salt, and pepper. Add the bay leaf and whisk to combine everything.
6. Cook on low for 6-8 hours or high for 4-5 hours until the meat is tender and the veggies are cooked.
7. Discard the bay leaf. Ladle the stew into bowl and top with fresh parsley.

Nutrition Information (Per Serving):

Calories: 320 Protein: 28g Carbohydrates: 12g Dietary Fiber: 4g Sugar: 5g Fat: 18g

Low-Carb Pork Chops with Garlic Mushrooms

Prep Time: 10 minutes Cook Time: 20 minutes Servings: 4

Ingredients:

- 4 boneless pork chops (about 1-inch thick)
- 2 tbsp olive oil (or avocado oil)
- 1 tsp sea salt
- 1/2 tsp black pepper
- 1/2 tsp smoked paprika
- 2 tbsp butter (or ghee)
- 3 cloves garlic, minced
- 8 ounces mushrooms (button or cremini), sliced
- 1/4 cup of chicken broth (low-sodium)
- 1/4 cup of heavy cream
- 1 tbsp fresh thyme leaves
- Fresh parsley, chopped (for garnish)

Instructions:

1. Pat the pork chops dry with a paper towel. Season each side with salt, pepper, and smoked paprika.
2. Heat 1 tbsp olive oil in a large pan over medium-high heat. Sear the pork chops for 3-4 minutes per side until golden brown and cooked through (internal temperature should be 145°F/63°C). Place the pork chops on a platter and cover with foil to keep warm.
3. Combine the remaining tbsp of olive oil and butter in the same skillet. Sauté the minced garlic for 30 seconds until aromatic.
4. Cook the sliced mushrooms for 4-5 minutes, turning periodically, until they are brown and soft.
5. Pour in the chicken broth and whisk to remove any browned pieces from the bottom of the skillet. If using, stir in the heavy cream and boil for 2-3 minutes until the sauce thickens slightly.
6. Stir in the thyme leaves, return the pork chops to the skillet, and spoon the mushroom sauce. To reheat the pork chops, cook for 1–2 minutes.
7. Plate the pork chops and top with the garlic mushroom sauce. Garnish with fresh parsley.

Nutrition Information (Per Serving):

Calories: 350 Protein: 28g Carbohydrates: 6g Dietary Fiber: 2g Sugar: 2g Fat: 24g

Sheet Pan Salmon & Veggies

Prep Time: 10 minutes Cook Time: 20 minutes Servings: 4

Ingredients:

- 4 salmon fillets (about 6 oz each)
- 1 pound asparagus, trimmed
- 1 red bell pepper, sliced
- 1 zucchini, sliced into rounds
- 1 red onion, sliced
- 2 tbsp olive oil
- 2 cloves garlic, minced
- 1 lemon, juiced and zested
- 1 tsp dried oregano
- 1/2 tsp smoked paprika
- 1/2 tsp sea salt
- 1/4 tsp black pepper
- Fresh parsley, chopped (for garnish)
- Lemon wedges (for serving)

Instructions:

1. Preheat the oven to 400 °F (200 °C). Line a large baking sheet with parchment or aluminium foil.
2. Place the asparagus, bell pepper slices, zucchini rounds, and red onion slices on a baking sheet. Drizzle with 1 tbsp olive oil and sprinkle with salt and pepper. Toss to coat evenly.
3. Combine the remaining tbsp olive oil, minced garlic, lemon juice, lemon zest, oregano, smoked paprika, salt, and pepper in a small bowl.
4. Place the salmon fillets on the baking sheet, nestled between the vegetables. Brush the salmon with the lemon-garlic mixture.
5. Bake for 15-20 minutes until the salmon is well cooked and readily flaked with a fork and the veggies are soft.
6. Garnish with fresh parsley and lemon wedges. Enjoy as hot.

Nutrition Information (Per Serving):

Calories: 350 Protein: 30g Carbohydrates: 10g Dietary Fiber: 3g Sugar: 4g Fat: 20g

Grilled Veggie & Chicken Kebabs

Prep Time: 20 minutes Cook Time: 15 minutes Servings: 4

Ingredients:

- 1 1/2 pounds boneless, skinless chicken breasts cut into 1-inch cubes
- 1 red bell pepper, cut into 1-inch pieces
- 1 yellow bell pepper, cut into 1-inch pieces
- 1 zucchini, sliced into 1/2-inch rounds
- 1 red onion, cut into wedges
- 1 cup of cherry tomatoes
- 2 tbsp olive oil
- 2 cloves garlic, minced
- Juice of 1 lemon
- 1 tbsp fresh parsley, chopped
- 1 tsp dried oregano
- 1 tsp smoked paprika
- 1/2 tsp ground cumin
- 1/2 tsp sea salt
- 1/4 tsp black pepper

Instructions:

1. Combine the olive oil, garlic, lemon juice, parsley, oregano, smoked paprika, cumin, salt, and black pepper in a large mixing bowl.
2. Toss the chicken cubes in the marinade to coat them uniformly. Cover and chill for at least 30 minutes (up to 2 hours for maximum taste).
3. Thread marinated chicken, bell peppers, zucchini, red onion, and cherry tomatoes onto skewers, alternating chicken and vegetables.
4. Preheat the grill over medium-high heat and gently oil the grates to avoid sticking.
5. Place the kebabs on the grill and cook for 12-15 minutes, flipping every 3-4 minutes, until the chicken is fully cooked (internal temperature should reach 165°F/74°C) and the vegetables are slightly browned.
6. Place the kebabs on a plate and top with more fresh parsley. Serve hot, with lemon slices on the side.

Nutrition Information (Per Serving):

Calories: 280 Protein: 28g Carbohydrates: 10g Dietary Fiber: 3g Sugar: 5g Fat: 14g

Eggplant Parmesan Casserole

Prep Time: 20 minutes

Cook Time: 40 minutes

Servings: 6

Ingredients:

- 2 medium eggplants, sliced into 1/4-inch rounds
- 2 tbsp olive oil
- 1 tsp sea salt
- 1/2 tsp black pepper
- 1 tsp dried oregano
- 1 tsp garlic powder
- 2 cups of marinara sauce (no added sugar)
- 1 cup of ricotta cheese
- 1 large egg
- 1 cup of shredded mozzarella cheese
- 1/2 cup of grated Parmesan cheese
- 1/4 cup of fresh basil leaves, chopped (for garnish)

Instructions:

1. Preheat the oven to 375° Fahrenheit (190° Celsius). Line a baking sheet with parchment paper.
2. Place the eggplant slices in a single layer on the baking sheet. Brush both sides with olive oil and season with salt, pepper, oregano, and garlic powder. Bake for 15 minutes, turning halfway through, until soft and lightly brown.
3. Blend the ricotta cheese and egg in a small bowl until thoroughly combined. Set aside.
4. Spread a thin layer of marinara sauce on the bottom of a 9x13-inch baking dish. Spread half of the roasted eggplant slices over the sauce. Spread half of the ricotta mixture over the eggplant, then add a layer of mozzarella and a sprinkle of Parmesan.
5. Repeat with the remaining eggplant, ricotta mixture, and cheese, ending with a layer of marinara sauce and a liberal sprinkling of mozzarella and Parmesan on top.
6. Cover the dish with aluminum foil and bake for 25 minutes. Remove the cover and bake for 10-15 more or until the cheese is melted and bubbling.
7. Allow the dish to cool for 5–10 minutes before serving. Garnish with fresh basil leaves.

Nutrition Information (Per Serving):

Calories: 290 Protein: 14g Carbohydrates: 15g Dietary Fiber: 6g Sugar: 8g

Thai Basil Chicken Stir-Fry

Prep Time: 10 minutes Cook Time: 15 minutes Servings: 4

Ingredients:

- 1 pound ground chicken
- 2 tbsp olive oil
- 4 cloves garlic, minced
- 2 Thai bird's eye chilies, finely chopped
- 1 small onion, thinly sliced
- 1 red bell pepper, sliced
- 2 cups of fresh basil leaves
- 3 tbsp low-sodium soy sauce
- 1 tbsp fish sauce
- 1 tbsp oyster sauce (optional)
- 1 tsp sweetener of choice
- Juice of 1 lime
- 1/4 tsp black pepper

Instructions:

1. In a large skillet or wok, heat the olive oil over medium-high. Combine the minced garlic and chopped chiles. Sauté for approximately 30 seconds until fragrant.
2. Add the ground chicken to the skillet. Break it up with a spatula and heat for 5-7 minutes or until browned and cooked.
3. Cook for 3-4 minutes, stirring in the chopped onion and bell pepper, until the veggies have softened somewhat.
4. In a small mixing bowl, combine the soy sauce, fish sauce, oyster sauce (if using), sugar, and lime juice. Pour the sauce over the chicken mixture and toss thoroughly to coat.
5. Add the fresh basil leaves and simmer for 1-2 minutes or until wilted. Stir thoroughly to incorporate all of the flavors.
6. Plate the stir-fry hot with cauliflower rice as a low-carb option. Garnish with more basil leaves and lime wedges.

Nutrition Information (Per Serving):

Calories: 250 Protein: 23g Carbohydrates: 8g Dietary Fiber: 2g Sugar: 3g

Lemon Pepper Tilapia with Steamed Greens

Prep Time: 10 minutes Cook Time: 15 minutes Servings: 4

Ingredients:

- For the Tilapia:
- 4 tilapia fillets (about 6 oz each)
- 2 tbsp olive oil
- Juice and zest of 1 lemon
- 1 tsp lemon pepper seasoning
- 1/2 tsp garlic powder
- 1/2 tsp sea salt
- 1/4 tsp black pepper
- 1 tbsp fresh parsley, chopped (for garnish)
- Lemon wedges (for serving)
- For the Steamed Greens:
- 2 cups of broccoli florets
- 2 cups of spinach leaves
- 1 tbsp olive oil
- 1 clove garlic, minced
- Pinch of sea salt
- Pinch of black pepper

Instructions:

1. Preheat the oven to 400 °F (200 °C). Cover a baking sheet with parchment paper or gently oil it.
2. Pat the fillets dry with a paper towel. Combine the olive oil, lemon juice, zest, lemon pepper spice, garlic powder, salt, and black pepper in a small mixing bowl.
3. Brush the spice mixture equally over both sides of the tilapia fillets before placing them on the prepared baking sheet.
4. Bake the tilapia for 10-12 minutes or until it is well cooked and readily flaked with a fork.
5. While the tilapia bakes, prepare the steamed greens: Heat 1 tbsp olive oil in a large pan over medium heat. Sauté the minced garlic for 30 seconds, until aromatic.
6. Cook the broccoli florets for 3-4 minutes, stirring occasionally. Add the spinach leaves, season with salt and pepper, and simmer for 2-3 minutes or until wilted.
7. Serve the cooked tilapia with steamed greens on the side. Garnish the fish with fresh parsley and serve with lemon wedges.

Nutrition Information (Per Serving):

Calories: 220 Protein: 28g Carbohydrates: 6g Dietary Fiber: 3g Sugar: 2g Fat: 10g

Low-Carb Lamb & Vegetable Curry

Prep Time: 15 minutes Cook Time: 45 minutes Servings: 4

Ingredients:

- 1 1/2 pounds lamb shoulder, cut into 1-inch cubes
- 2 tbsp coconut oil (or olive oil)
- 1 medium onion, diced
- 3 cloves garlic, minced
- 1-inch piece of ginger, grated
- 2 tbsp curry powder
- 1 tsp ground cumin
- 1 tsp ground coriander
- 1/2 tsp turmeric powder
- 1/2 tsp chili powder (optional, for spice)
- 1 can (14 oz) coconut milk (full-fat)
- 1/2 cup of beef broth
- 1 small eggplant, diced
- 1 red bell pepper, diced
- 1 zucchini, sliced
- 2 cups of fresh spinach leaves
- 1 tsp sea salt
- 1/2 tsp black pepper
- Juice of 1 lime
- Fresh cilantro, chopped (for garnish)

Instructions:

1. In a large saucepan or Dutch oven, melt the coconut oil over medium-high heat. Add the lamb cubes and sear on both sides for 5-7 minutes or until browned. Remove the lamb from the saucepan and put it aside.
2. Combine the chopped onion, minced garlic, and grated ginger in the same saucepan. Sauté for 3-4 minutes, until softened and aromatic.
3. Combine the curry powder, cumin, coriander, turmeric, and chili powder (if using). Cook for one minute, stirring constantly to toast the spices.

4. Pour in the coconut milk and beef broth, scraping off any browned pieces on the bottom of the saucepan. Heat the mixture to a simmer.
5. Return the seared meat to the pot. Combine the eggplant, bell pepper, and zucchini. Stir well to mix. Season with salt and black pepper.
6. Cover the saucepan and simmer for 30-35 minutes, stirring regularly, until the lamb is tender and the veggies are fully cooked.
7. Stir in the spinach leaves and simmer for 2-3 minutes or until wilted. Add the lime juice and season as required.
8. Ladle the curry into bowls and top with fresh cilantro. Serve and enjoy.

Nutrition Information (Per Serving):

Calories: 380 Protein: 28g Carbohydrates: 12g Dietary Fiber: 4g Sugar: 5g Fat: 25g

Spicy Cauliflower & Chicken Skillet

Prep Time: 10 minutes Cook Time: 20 minutes Servings: 4

Ingredients:

- 1 pound boneless, skinless chicken breast, diced
- 2 tbsp olive oil (or avocado oil)
- 1 medium onion, diced
- 3 cloves garlic, minced
- 1 medium head of cauliflower, cut into small florets
- 1 red bell pepper, diced
- 1 jalapeño, finely chopped
- 1 tsp smoked paprika
- 1 tsp ground cumin
- 1/2 tsp chili powder
- 1/4 tsp cayenne pepper
- 1/2 tsp sea salt
- 1/4 tsp black pepper
- 1/4 cup of chicken broth (low-sodium)
- Juice of 1 lime
- 1/4 cup of fresh cilantro, chopped

Instructions:

1. In a large pan, warm 1 tbsp olive oil over medium-high heat. Season the chopped chicken breast with salt and pepper. Sauté for 5-7 minutes or until the chicken is browned and thoroughly cooked. Remove the chicken from the skillet and put it aside.
2. In the same skillet, heat the remaining tbsp olive oil. Combine diced onion, minced garlic, and jalapeño. Cook for 2-3 minutes, until aromatic.
3. Place the cauliflower florets and red bell pepper in the skillet. Season with smoked paprika, ground cumin, chili powder, and cayenne pepper (optional). Stir well to coat the veggies with the seasonings.
4. Pour in the chicken broth and whisk to remove any browned pieces from the bottom of the skillet. Cover and heat for 5-7 minutes or until the cauliflower is soft.
5. Return the cooked chicken to the skillet and stir well. Squeeze the lime juice over the **dish** and simmer for 1-2 minutes until well cooked.
6. Garnish with fresh cilantro and serve hot.

Nutrition Information (Per Serving):

Calories: 280 Protein: 28g Carbohydrates: 10g Dietary Fiber: 4g Sugar: 4g Fat: 14g

CHAPTER 6: SNACKS AND SIDES

Guacamole & Veggie Sticks

Prep Time: 10 minutes Servings: 4

Ingredients:

- For the Guacamole:
- 3 ripe avocados
- 1 small red onion, finely diced
- 1 medium tomato, diced
- 1 jalapeño, finely chopped (remove seeds for less heat)
- 2 cloves garlic, minced
- Juice of 1 lime
- 1/4 cup of fresh cilantro, chopped
- 1/2 tsp sea salt
- 1/4 tsp black pepper
- 1/4 tsp cumin (optional)
- For the Veggie Sticks:
- 2 large carrots, cut into sticks
- 2 celery stalks, cut into sticks
- 1 red bell pepper, sliced into strips
- 1 cucumber, sliced into sticks

Instructions:

1. Cut the avocados in half, remove the pits, and scoop the flesh into a large bowl. Mash the avocados with a fork until smooth or chunky, according to your preference.
2. Combine diced onion, tomato, jalapeño, minced garlic, lime juice, and cilantro with the mashed avocado. Stir well to mix.
3. Season the guacamole with salt, pepper, and cumin (optional). Season to taste.
4. Place the carrot sticks, celery sticks, bell pepper strips, and cucumber sticks on a serving plate.
5. Transfer the guacamole to a serving bowl and arrange in the center of the plate. Enjoy the guacamole with fresh vegetable sticks.

Nutrition Information (Per Serving):

Calories: 180 Protein: 3g Carbohydrates: 15g Dietary Fiber: 8g Sugar: 5g Fat: 14g

Baked Zucchini Fries

Prep Time: 15 minutes

Cook Time: 20 minutes

Servings: 4

Ingredients:

- 2 medium zucchinis
- 1/2 cup of almond flour
- 1/4 cup of grated Parmesan cheese (optional)
- 1 tsp garlic powder
- 1 tsp smoked paprika
- 1/2 tsp sea salt
- 1/4 tsp black pepper
- 2 large eggs
- Olive oil spray (for baking)

Instructions:

1. Preheat the oven to 425° Fahrenheit (220° Celsius). Cover a baking sheet with parchment paper or gently oil it.
2. Cut the zucchini into thin, fry-like sticks about 1/4 inch thick. In a small bowl, whisk the eggs until thoroughly combined.
3. In another bowl, mix the almond flour, Parmesan cheese (if using), garlic powder, smoky paprika, salt, and black pepper.
4. Dip each zucchini stick into the egg mixture, then roll in the almond flour mixture, pressing gently to coat.
5. Arrange the coated zucchini sticks on the prepared baking sheet in a single layer. Spray the tops gently with olive oil.
6. Bake the fries for 18-20 minutes, flipping halfway through, until golden brown and crispy.
7. Serve the zucchini fries hot with your favorite low-carb dipping sauce, such as marinara or garlic aioli.

Nutrition Information (Per Serving):

Calories: 150 Protein: 6g Carbohydrates: 8g Dietary Fiber: 4g Sugar: 3g Fat: 11g

Deviled Eggs with Avocado

Prep Time: 15 minutes Cook Time: 10 minutes Servings: 4

Ingredients:

- 4 large eggs
- 1 ripe avocado
- 1 tbsp mayonnaise
- 1 tsp Dijon mustard
- Juice of 1/2 lime
- 1/4 tsp sea salt
- 1/4 tsp black pepper
- 1/4 tsp garlic powder
- 1 tbsp fresh cilantro, chopped (for garnish)
- Paprika (for garnish)

Instructions:

1. Put the eggs in a pot and cover with water. Bring to a boil over medium-high heat. Once boiling, reduce the heat to a simmer for 10 minutes. Let the eggs cool in a bowl of cold water for 5 minutes.
2. Once cold, peel and cut the eggs in half lengthwise. Carefully scoop off the yolks and transfer them to a mixing bowl.
3. Using a fork, mash the egg yolks and avocado until smooth. Mix in mayonnaise, Dijon mustard, lime juice, salt, pepper, and garlic powder. Mix well to mix.
4. Spoon or pipe the avocado mixture back into the egg white halves.
5. Season with paprika and fresh cilantro. Serve immediately.

Nutrition Information (Per Serving - 2 halves):

Calories: 120 Protein: 6g Carbohydrates: 3g Dietary Fiber: 2g Sugar: 0g Fat: 10g

Greek Yogurt Ranch Dip with Cucumbers

Prep Time: 10 minutes Servings: 4

Ingredients:

- For the Ranch Dip:
- 1 cup of plain Greek yogurt
- 1 tbsp fresh dill, finely chopped
- 1 tbsp fresh parsley, finely chopped
- 1 tsp garlic powder
- 1 tsp onion powder
- 1/2 tsp dried chives
- 1/2 tsp sea salt
- 1/4 tsp black pepper
- Juice of 1/2 lemon
- 1-2 tbsp water (to thin, if needed)
- For the Dippers:
- 2 large cucumbers, sliced into rounds or sticks

Instructions:

1. In a medium bowl, mix the Greek yogurt, dill, parsley, garlic powder, onion powder, dried chives, salt, and black pepper.
2. Add the lemon juice and blend thoroughly. Add 1-2 tsp water for consistency if the dip is too thick.
3. Taste and adjust the seasoning as required. Refrigerate for at least 10 minutes to enable the flavors to mingle.
4. Transfer the dip to a serving dish and arrange the cucumber slices around it. Enjoy as a nutritious, low-carb snack.

Nutrition Information (Per Serving):

Calories: 70 Protein: 6g Carbohydrates: 4g Dietary Fiber: 1g Sugar: 3g Fat: 2g

Low-Carb Cheese & Meat Platter

Prep Time: 15 minutes

Servings: 6

Ingredients:

- Cheeses:
- 6 oz sharp cheddar cheese, sliced
- 6 oz mozzarella cheese, sliced or in bite-sized cubes
- 4 oz blue cheese or goat cheese
- Meats:
- 6 oz prosciutto, thinly sliced
- 6 oz salami, sliced
- 4 oz smoked turkey or roast beef, sliced
- Low-Carb Additions:
- 1/2 cup of olives (Kalamata or green), pitted
- 1/2 cup of cherry tomatoes
- 1/2 cup of roasted nuts
- 1/2 cup of pickles or pickled vegetables
- 1 small cucumber, sliced into rounds
- 1/4 cup of Dijon mustard or whole-grain mustard (for dipping)
- Fresh herbs for garnish

Instructions:

1. Divide the cheese slices and cubes into pieces on a large serving board or tray. Fold the prosciutto, salami, and smoked turkey into rolls or fans and arrange them alongside the cheese.
2. Fill the holes with olives, cherry tomatoes, toasted almonds, pickles, and cucumber slices. Place a small bowl of Dijon mustard on the side for dipping.
3. To add a decorative touch, garnish the tray with fresh herbs. Serve immediately.

Nutrition Information (Per Serving):

Calories: 280 Protein: 16g Carbohydrates: 4g Dietary Fiber: 1g Sugar: 2g Fat: 22g

Spicy Roasted Chickpeas

Prep Time: 5 minutes

Cook Time: 30-35 minutes

Servings: 4

Ingredients:

- 1 can (15 oz) chickpeas, drained and rinsed
- 1 tbsp olive oil
- 1 tsp smoked paprika
- 1/2 tsp chili powder
- 1/2 tsp cumin
- 1/4 tsp cayenne pepper (optional for extra spice)
- 1/2 tsp garlic powder
- 1/2 tsp sea salt
- 1/4 tsp black pepper

Instructions:

1. Preheat the oven to 400 °F (200 °C). Line a baking sheet with parchment paper.
2. Using a paper towel, thoroughly dry the chickpeas. This will allow them to cook evenly and get crispy.
3. In a bowl, combine the chickpeas, olive oil, smoked paprika, chili powder, cumin, cayenne pepper, garlic powder, salt, and black pepper. Mix well to coat the chickpeas evenly.
4. Place the seasoned chickpeas in a single layer on the prepared baking sheet. Roast for 30-35 minutes, stirring the pan halfway through, until the chickpeas turn golden and crispy.
5. Allow the chickpeas to cool for five minutes before serving. Serve and enjoy.

Nutrition Information (Per Serving):

Calories: 120 Protein: 5g Carbohydrates: 18g Dietary Fiber: 5g Sugar: 1g Fat: 4g

Broccoli Cheddar Bites

Prep Time: 15 minutes

Cook Time: 20 minutes

Servings: 4 (12 bites)

Ingredients:

- 2 cups of broccoli florets, finely chopped
- 1 cup of shredded cheddar cheese
- 1/2 cup of almond flour
- 2 large eggs
- 1/4 cup of grated Parmesan cheese
- 1 tsp garlic powder
- 1/2 tsp smoked paprika
- 1/2 tsp sea salt
- 1/4 tsp black pepper
- Olive oil spray (for baking)

Instructions:

1. Preheat the oven to 375° Fahrenheit (190° Celsius). Line a baking sheet with parchment paper and gently coat it with olive oil.
2. Steam the chopped broccoli in a microwave-safe bowl until soft, about 2-3 minutes. Allow to cool somewhat, then wipe dry with a paper towel to eliminate extra moisture.
3. Add steamed broccoli, cheddar cheese, almond flour, eggs, Parmesan cheese, garlic powder, smoky paprika, salt, and black pepper in a large mixing bowl. Mix well until the ingredients are uniformly distributed.
4. Scoop approximately 1-2 tsp. of the mixture and shape into little, bite-sized balls. Place them on the prepared baking sheet.
5. Spray the tops of the bits liberally with olive oil and bake for 18-20 minutes or until golden brown and crispy on the exterior.
6. Allow the bites to cool slightly before serving.

Nutrition Information (Per Serving - 3 bites):

Calories: 150 Protein: 8g Carbohydrates: 5g Dietary Fiber: 2g Sugar: 1g Fat: 10g

Almond-Crusted Mozzarella Sticks

Prep Time: 15 minutes

Cook Time: 10 minutes

Servings: 4

Ingredients:

- 8 mozzarella string cheese sticks, halved
- 1/2 cup of almond flour
- 1/4 cup of grated Parmesan cheese
- 1 tsp garlic powder
- 1 tsp Italian seasoning
- 1/2 tsp smoked paprika
- 1/4 tsp sea salt
- 1/4 tsp black pepper
- 2 large eggs, beaten
- Olive oil spray (for baking)
- For Serving:
- 1/2 cup of marinara sauce (low-carb, for dipping)

Instructions:

1. Cut each mozzarella stick in half, resulting in 16 pieces. Place the cheese sticks on a bowl and freeze for at least an hour.
2. Preheat the oven to 400 °F (200 °C). Line a baking sheet with parchment paper and gently coat it with olive oil.
3. Beat the eggs in one bowl. Combine the almond flour, Parmesan cheese, garlic powder, Italian spice, smoked paprika, salt, and black pepper in another bowl.
4. Dip each frozen cheese stick in the egg, then roll in the almond flour mixture, pressing lightly to achieve uniform coverage. Repeat the process twice for even more crunch.
5. Place the coated mozzarella sticks on the prepared baking sheet. Lightly spray the tops with olive oil. Bake for 8–10 minutes, turning halfway through, until golden brown and crispy.
6. Allow the mozzarella sticks to cool slightly before serving. Enjoy with warm marinara sauce for dipping.

Nutrition Information (Per Serving - 4 sticks):

Calories: 220 Protein: 12g Carbohydrates: 5g Dietary Fiber: 2g Sugar: 1g Fat: 17g

Keto Cauliflower Hummus

Prep Time: 10 minutes

Cook Time: 10 minutes

Servings: 6

Ingredients:

- 1 medium head of cauliflower, cut into florets
- 2 tbsp olive oil
- 2 cloves garlic, minced
- 1/4 cup of tahini
- 2 tbsp lemon juice
- 1/2 tsp ground cumin
- 1/2 tsp smoked paprika
- 1/2 tsp sea salt
- 1/4 tsp black pepper
- 2 tbsp water (to thin, if needed)
- Fresh parsley, chopped (for garnish)

Instructions:

1. Heat a pot of water to a boil. Add the cauliflower florets and cook for 8-10 minutes, until very soft. Drain and cool gently.
2. Mix the steamed cauliflower, olive oil, garlic, tahini, lemon juice, cumin, smoked paprika, salt, and black pepper in a food processor. Blend until smooth and creamy. If the mixture is too thick, add 1-2 tsp water and combine until the required consistency is achieved.
3. Taste and season with extra salt, lemon juice, or paprika if necessary.
4. Transfer the hummus to a serving bowl. Drizzle with olive oil, season with smoky paprika, and serve with fresh parsley.
5. Serve with low-carb dippers such as cucumber slices, bell pepper strips, and celery sticks.

Nutrition Information (Per Serving):

Calories: 80 Protein: 3g Carbohydrates: 6g Dietary Fiber: 2g Sugar: 2g Fat: 6g

Celery Sticks with Nut Butter

Prep Time: 5 minutes

Servings: 2

Ingredients:

- 4 large celery stalks, trimmed and cut into 3-inch pieces
- 1/4 cup of almond butter
- 1/4 tsp cinnamon
- 1 tbsp chia seeds or crushed nuts
- A pinch of sea salt (optional for a savory touch)

Instructions:

1. Wash the celery stalks thoroughly before cutting them into 3-inch sticks.
2. Spread roughly 1 tbsp nut butter on each celery stick.
3. To add crunch and flavor, sprinkle cinnamon, chia seeds, or crumbled nuts on top, for a savory taste, season with a sprinkle of sea salt.
4. Place the celery sticks on a plate and eat.

Nutrition Information (Per Serving):

Calories: 150 Protein: 5g Carbohydrates: 7g Dietary Fiber: 4g Sugar: 2g Fat: 13g

Bell Pepper Nachos with Ground Turkey

Prep Time: 15 minutes Cook Time: 15 minutes Servings: 4

Ingredients:

- 3 large bell peppers, cut into bite-sized triangles
- 1 tbsp olive oil
- 1 pound ground turkey
- 1 small onion, diced
- 2 cloves garlic, minced
- 1 tsp chili powder
- 1/2 tsp cumin
- 1/2 tsp smoked paprika
- 1/2 tsp sea salt
- 1/4 tsp black pepper
- 1/2 cup of shredded cheddar cheese
- 1/4 cup of diced tomatoes
- 1/4 cup of sliced black olives (optional)
- 1/4 cup of fresh cilantro, chopped
- 1 jalapeño, sliced
- 1/4 cup of sour cream (optional)
- 1/4 cup of guacamole (optional)

Instructions:

1. Preheat the oven to 375° Fahrenheit (190° Celsius). Line a large baking sheet with parchment paper.
2. Place the bell pepper triangles in a single layer on the prepared baking sheet.
3. In a large skillet, heat olive oil over medium heat. Sauté the diced onion for 3-4 minutes, until softened. Add the minced garlic and cook for a further 30 seconds.
4. Add the ground turkey to the skillet and mix it with a spatula. Cook for 5-7 minutes, until browned and heated through.
5. Season the turkey with chili powder, cumin, smoked paprika, salt, and black pepper. Stir thoroughly and simmer for another 2 minutes. Remove from heat.
6. Distribute the seasoned ground turkey equally among the bell pepper slices. Sprinkle with grated cheese.
7. Place the nachos in the oven for 8-10 minutes or until the cheese melts and bubbles.
8. Garnish with chopped tomatoes, black olives, fresh cilantro, and sliced jalapeños (optional). Serve hot, with sour cream and guacamole on the side.

Nutrition Information (Per Serving):

Calories: 250 Protein: 20g Carbohydrates: 10g Dietary Fiber: 3g Sugar: 4g Fat: 14g

Stuffed Mushrooms with Spinach & Feta

Prep Time: 15 minutes Cook Time: 20 minutes Servings: 4

Ingredients:

- 16 large white or cremini mushrooms, stems removed
- 1 tbsp olive oil
- 2 cloves garlic, minced
- 2 cups of fresh spinach, chopped
- 1/4 cup of onion, finely diced
- 1/2 cup of crumbled feta cheese
- 1/4 cup of cream cheese, softened
- 1/4 tsp sea salt
- 1/4 tsp black pepper
- 1/2 tsp dried oregano
- 1/4 cup of grated Parmesan cheese
- Fresh parsley, chopped (for garnish)

Instructions:

1. Preheat the oven to 375° Fahrenheit (190° Celsius). Line a baking sheet with parchment paper.
2. Clean the mushrooms with a moist paper towel and remove the stems. Place the mushroom caps on the prepared baking sheet.
3. Heat the olive oil in a medium-sized pan. Sauté the onion for 2-3 minutes, until softened. Add the minced garlic and cook for a further 30 seconds.
4. Add the chopped spinach and simmer for 2-3 minutes or until wilted. Remove from heat and allow it to cool slightly.
5. Add the sautéed spinach, feta cheese, cream cheese, salt, pepper, and oregano to a mixing bowl. Mix well until creamy.
6. Spoon the spinach and feta filling into each mushroom cap, pushing gently. If desired, sprinkle the tops with grated Parmesan cheese.
7. Place the stuffed mushrooms in a warm oven and bake for 15-20 minutes or until soft and golden brown on top.
8. Garnish with fresh parsley and serve warm.

Nutrition Information (Per Serving - 4 mushrooms):

Calories: 120 Protein: 5g Carbohydrates: 5g Dietary Fiber: 2g Sugar: 2g Fat: 9g

Lemon & Garlic Roasted Asparagus

Prep Time: 5 minutes Cook Time: 15 minutes Servings: 4

Ingredients:

- 1 pound asparagus, trimmed
- 2 tbsp olive oil
- 2 cloves garlic, minced
- Zest of 1 lemon
- Juice of 1/2 lemon
- 1/2 tsp sea salt
- 1/4 tsp black pepper
- 1/4 tsp red pepper flakes
- Fresh parsley, chopped (for garnish)
- Lemon wedges (for serving)

Instructions:

1. Preheat the oven to 400 °F (200 °C). Cover a baking sheet with parchment paper or gently oil it.
2. Place the asparagus stalks in a single layer on the baking sheet. Drizzle with olive oil and season with minced garlic, lemon zest, salt, pepper, and red pepper flakes (if using).
3. Place the baking sheet in the oven and roast for 12-15 minutes or until the asparagus is tender and slightly browned.
4. Remove the asparagus from the oven and immediately sprinkle it with lemon juice. Toss lightly to coat.
5. Transfer the roasted asparagus to a serving plate. Garnish with fresh parsley and serve alongside additional lemon wedges.

Nutrition Information (Per Serving):

Calories: 80 Protein: 2g Carbohydrates: 5g Dietary Fiber: 2g Sugar: 2g Fat: 7g

Cucumber & Avocado Rolls

Prep Time: 15 minutes

Servings: 4 (8 rolls)

Ingredients:

- 1 large cucumber
- 1 ripe avocado
- 1 tbsp lemon juice
- 1/4 tsp sea salt
- 1/4 tsp black pepper
- 1 tbsp fresh chives, chopped
- 1 tbsp fresh cilantro or parsley, chopped
- 1/4 cup of cream cheese
- 1 tbsp sesame seeds (for garnish)
- Soy sauce or tamari (for dipping, optional)

Instructions:

1. Cut the cucumber lengthwise into thin, broad strips using a mandoline or vegetable peeler. Dry the strips with a paper towel to eliminate excess moisture.
2. In a mixing bowl, mash the avocado with a fork until smooth. Combine lemon juice, sea salt, black pepper, chives, and cilantro. Mix thoroughly. If using, fold in the cream cheese for extra richness.
3. Place a cucumber strip flat on a chopping board. Spread a thin coating of the avocado mixture across one end of the strip. Roll the cucumber firmly around the filling.
4. Sprinkle sesame seeds on the rolls.
5. Arrange the cucumber and avocado wraps on a serving platter. Serve as a pleasant, low-carb appetizer or snack. If preferred, serve with dipping sauces such as soy sauce or tamari.

Nutrition Information (Per Serving - 2 rolls):

Calories: 80 Protein: 1g Carbohydrates: 5g Dietary Fiber: 3g Sugar: 1g Fat: 7g

Mini Caprese Salad Skewers

Prep Time: 10 minutes

Servings: 4 (12 skewers)

Ingredients:

- 12 cherry tomatoes
- 12 fresh mozzarella balls
- 12 fresh basil leaves
- 2 tbsp olive oil
- 1 tbsp balsamic vinegar (optional)
- 1/4 tsp sea salt
- 1/4 tsp black pepper
- Wooden toothpicks or small skewers

Instructions:

1. Thread one cherry tomato, mozzarella ball, and basil leaf onto a toothpick or short skewer.
2. Place the skewers on a serving plate. Drizzle with olive oil and balsamic vinegar (optional).
3. Season the skewers with sea salt and black pepper.
4. Enjoy the skewers as a light, refreshing appetizer or snack.

Nutrition Information (Per Serving - 3 skewers):

Calories: 120 Protein: 6g Carbohydrates: 4g Dietary Fiber: 1g Sugar: 2g Fat: 10g

Baked Brussels Sprouts Chips

Prep Time: 10 minutes

Cook Time: 15 minutes

Servings: 4

Ingredients:

- 1 pound Brussels sprouts
- 2 tbsp olive oil
- 1/2 tsp sea salt
- 1/4 tsp black pepper
- 1/4 tsp garlic powder
- 1/4 tsp smoked paprika

Instructions:

1. Preheat the oven to 400 °F (200 °C). Line a baking sheet with parchment paper.
2. Trim the ends of the Brussels sprouts and gently remove the outer leaves. Continue peeling until you have a bowl of leaves (save the cores for another use).
3. In a large mixing bowl, combine the Brussels sprout leaves, olive oil, salt, pepper, garlic powder, and smoky paprika (if using).
4. Place the seasoned leaves in a single layer on the prepared baking sheet.
5. Roast in the oven for 10-15 minutes, tossing halfway through or until the leaves are crispy and lightly browned.
6. Remove from the oven and allow it to cool slightly. Serve and enjoy.

Nutrition Information (Per Serving):

Calories: 80 Protein: 2g Carbohydrates: 6g Dietary Fiber: 3g Sugar: 1g

Spiced Cauliflower Popcorn

Prep Time: 10 minutes

Cook Time: 25 minutes

Servings: 4

Ingredients:

- 1 medium head of cauliflower, cut into small bite-sized florets
- 2 tbsp olive oil
- 1 tsp smoked paprika
- 1 tsp ground cumin
- 1/2 tsp garlic powder
- 1/4 tsp chili powder
- 1/2 tsp sea salt
- 1/4 tsp black pepper

Instructions:

1. Preheat the oven to 400 °F (200 °C). Line a baking sheet with parchment paper.
2. Cut cauliflower into tiny, bite-sized florets that resemble popcorn bits.
3. In a large mixing bowl, combine the cauliflower florets, olive oil, smoked paprika, cumin, garlic powder, chili powder (if using), sea salt, and black pepper. Mix thoroughly to coat the cauliflower evenly.
4. Place the seasoned cauliflower in a single layer on the prepared baking sheet. Roast for 20-25 minutes, stirring halfway through, or until the cauliflower is golden brown and crispy on the edges.
5. Allow the cauliflower popcorn to cool slightly before consuming. Serve warm.

Nutrition Information (Per Serving):

Calories: 90 Protein: 2g Carbohydrates: 7g Dietary Fiber: 3g Sugar: 2g Fat: 6g

Turkey & Cheese Roll-Ups

Prep Time: 5 minutes

Servings: 4

Ingredients:

- 8 slices deli turkey breast
- 8 slices cheese
- 1/4 cup of cream cheese, softened
- 1 tbsp Dijon mustard (optional)
- 1/2 tsp garlic powder
- 1/2 tsp smoked paprika
- 1/4 cup of fresh spinach leaves (or arugula)
- Toothpicks (for securing)

Instructions:

1. Combine the cream cheese, Dijon mustard, garlic powder, and smoked paprika in a small bowl.
2. Place a piece of turkey flat on a chopping board. Spread a thin layer of cream cheese mixture on top.
3. Top the turkey with a piece of cheese and a few spinach leaves.
4. Starting at one end, firmly roll up the turkey and cheese slices. If necessary, use a toothpick to secure the roll-up.
5. Arrange the roll-ups on a plate and serve immediately.

Nutrition Information (Per Serving - 2 roll-ups):

Calories: 150 Protein: 12g Carbohydrates: 2g Dietary Fiber: 0g Sugar: 1g Fat: 10g

Keto-Friendly Trail Mix

Prep Time: 5 minutes

Servings: 8

Ingredients:

- 1 cup of raw almonds
- 1/2 cup of raw pecans
- 1/2 cup of raw walnuts
- 1/4 cup of pumpkin seeds (pepitas)
- 1/4 cup of sunflower seeds
- 1/4 cup of unsweetened coconut flakes
- 1/4 cup of sugar-free dark chocolate chips
- 1/4 cup of freeze-dried raspberries or blueberries
- 1/2 tsp sea salt
- 1/2 tsp ground cinnamon

Instructions:

1. In a large mixing bowl, add almonds, pecans, walnuts, pumpkin seeds, sunflower seeds, coconut flakes, and chocolate chips (if using). If desired, add freeze-dried berries.
2. Sprinkle with sea salt and ground cinnamon, and toss to mix.
3. Transfer the trail mix to an airtight jar. Serve and enjoy.

Nutrition Information (Per Serving):

Calories: 200 Protein: 5g Carbohydrates: 6g Dietary Fiber: 3g Sugar: 1g Fat: 18g

Sautéed Garlic Green Beans

Prep Time: 5 minutes

Cook Time: 10 minutes

Servings: 4

Ingredients:

- 1 pound fresh green beans, trimmed
- 2 tbsp olive oil (or avocado oil)
- 3 cloves garlic, minced
- 1/2 tsp sea salt
- 1/4 tsp black pepper
- 1/4 tsp red pepper flakes
- Juice of 1/2 lemon
- 1 tbsp fresh parsley, chopped (for garnish)

Instructions:

1. Heat a large saucepan of water to a boil. Cook the green beans for 2-3 minutes until they turn bright green. Drain immediately and place in a bowl of cold water to halt the cooking process. Drain well before sautéing.
2. In a large pan, heat the olive oil over medium-high heat. Sauté the minced garlic for 30 seconds, until aromatic.
3. Add the green beans to the pan and season with salt, black pepper, and red pepper flakes (if using). Toss well to coat the beans with garlic and spices.
4. Sauté the green beans for 5-7 minutes, turning periodically until tender-crisp and gently browned.
5. Remove the heat and sprinkle with lemon juice for a bright, refreshing taste. Place on a serving plate and top with chopped parsley. Serve hot.

Nutrition Information (Per Serving):

Calories: 90 Protein: 2g Carbohydrates: 7g Dietary Fiber: 3g Fat: 7g

CHAPTER 7: DESSERT RECIPES

Almond Flour Chocolate Chip Cookies

Prep Time: 10 minutes Cook Time: 12-15 minutes Servings: 12 cookies

Ingredients:

- 2 cups of almond flour
- 1/4 cup of coconut oil melted
- 1/4 cup of granulated erythritol or monk fruit sweetener
- 1 large egg
- 1 tsp vanilla extract
- 1/2 tsp baking soda
- 1/4 tsp sea salt
- 1/2 cup of sugar-free dark chocolate chips

Instructions:

1. Preheat the oven to 350° Fahrenheit (175° Celsius). Line a baking sheet with parchment paper.
2. Blend the melted coconut oil, erythritol, egg, and vanilla extract in a large mixing bowl until thoroughly combined.
3. Add the almond flour, baking soda, and sea salt to the wet ingredients. Stir until dough forms.
4. Gently stir the sugar-free chocolate chips until they are equally distributed throughout the dough.
5. Scoop roughly 1 tbsp of dough for each cookie and shape it into a ball. Place the balls on the prepared baking sheet, spaced approximately 2 inches apart. Flatten each ball gently with your palm or a spoon.
6. Bake the cookies in the oven for 12-15 minutes or until golden brown around the edges.
7. Allow the cookies to cool on the baking sheet for 10 minutes before moving to a wire rack to finish cooling.

Nutrition Information (Per Cookie):

Calories: 130 Protein: 3g Carbohydrates: 6g Dietary Fiber: 2g Sugar: 1g Fat: 11g

Keto Vanilla Mug Cake

Prep Time: 2 minutes

Cook Time: 1-2 minutes

Servings: 1

Ingredients:

- 1/4 cup of almond flour
- 1 tbsp coconut flour
- 1/2 tsp baking powder
- 1 1/2 tbsp granulated erythritol or monk fruit sweetener
- 1 large egg
- 2 tbsp unsweetened almond milk
- 1 tbsp melted butter (or coconut oil)
- 1/2 tsp vanilla extract
- Pinch of sea salt

Instructions:

1. Mix the almond flour, coconut flour, baking powder, sweetener, and salt in a microwave-safe cup. Stir thoroughly to eliminate any lumps.
2. Combine the egg, almond milk, melted butter, and vanilla extract in the mug. Mix vigorously until the batter is smooth.
3. Microwave the cup on high for 1–2 minutes. Begin checking at the 1-minute mark. The cake is done when it has risen and settled in the center.
4. Allow the cup of cake to cool for a minute before serving. Optional toppings include a dollop of sugar-free whipped cream and a sprinkling of cinnamon.

Nutrition Information (Per Serving):

Calories: 220 Protein: 7g Carbohydrates: 6g Dietary Fiber: 3g Sugar: 1g Fat: 18g

Low-Carb Cheesecake Bites

Prep Time: 15 minutes

Servings: 12 bites

Ingredients:

- 8 oz cream cheese, softened
- 1/4 cup of powdered erythritol or monk fruit sweetener
- 1/4 cup of heavy cream
- 1 tsp vanilla extract
- 1 tbsp lemon juice
- 1/4 cup of almond flour
- 1 tbsp melted butter
- Topping Ideas (optional):
- Fresh berries
- Sugar-free chocolate chips
- Shredded unsweetened coconut

Instructions:

1. In a small bowl, combine the almond flour and melted butter. Place about 1 tsp of the mixture in the bottom of each tiny muffin cup of the silicone mold. Set aside.
2. An electric mixer smoothly the cream cheese in a medium mixing bowl. Combine the powdered sweetener, heavy cream, vanilla extract, and lemon juice. Mix until the filling is creamy and well-mixed.
3. Spoon the cheesecake mixture equally into the small muffin cups or silicone molds, filling them to the top.
4. Place the cheesecake pieces in the fridge for an hour to firm up.
5. Gently remove the cheesecake bits from the moulds and sprinkle them with fresh berries, chocolate chips, or shredded coconut.

Nutrition Information

Calories: 80 Protein: 2g Carbohydrates: 2g Dietary Fiber: 0g Sugar: 0g Fat: 8g

Chocolate Avocado Mousse

Prep Time: 5 minutes

Servings: 4

Ingredients:

- 2 ripe avocados
- 1/4 cup of unsweetened cocoa powder
- 1/4 cup of powdered erythritol or monk fruit sweetener
- 1/4 cup of unsweetened almond milk
- 1 tsp vanilla extract
- 1/8 tsp sea salt
- 1 tbsp coconut oil
- 1-2 tbsp sugar-free dark chocolate chips
- Fresh berries or mint leaves

Instructions:

1. In a food processor or blender, mix avocados, cocoa powder, sweetener, almond milk, vanilla extract, sea salt, and coconut oil (if using). Blend until smooth and creamy, scraping the sides as necessary.
2. Taste the mousse and add additional sweetness if necessary. Blend again to integrate.
3. Transfer the mousse to individual serving bowls or ramekins. Refrigerate for at least 30 minutes to let the flavors combine.
4. Garnish with sugar-free dark chocolate chips, fresh berries, or a sprig of mint. Serve cold.

Nutrition Information (Per Serving):

Calories: 180 Protein: 3g Carbohydrates: 10g Dietary Fiber: 6g Sugar: 1g Fat: 16g

Keto Coconut Macaroons

Prep Time: 10 minutes

Cook Time: 15-18 minutes

Servings: 12 macaroons

Ingredients:

- 2 cups of unsweetened shredded coconut
- 2 large egg whites
- 1/4 cup of granulated erythritol or monk fruit sweetener
- 1 tsp vanilla extract
- 1/4 tsp sea salt
- 1 tbsp coconut flour
- 2 tbsp sugar-free dark chocolate chips

Instructions:

1. Preheat the oven to 350° Fahrenheit (175° Celsius). Line a baking sheet with parchment paper.
2. Add the egg whites, sweetener, vanilla extract, and sea salt in a large mixing bowl. Whisk until thoroughly blended and foamy.
3. Incorporate the shredded coconut (and coconut flour, if using) into the egg-white mixture. Stir until the coconut is well covered and the mixture holds together.
4. Using a tbsp. scoop out tiny mounds of the mixture and set them on the prepared baking sheet, about 1 inch apart.
5. Bake for 15-18 minutes until the edges turn golden brown. Watch them closely as they brown fast at the finish.
6. Let the macaroons cool on the baking sheet for 5 minutes before transferring to a wire rack to finish cooling. If desired, melt the sugar-free chocolate chips and sprinkle them over the cooled macaroons.
7. Serve and enjoy.

Nutrition Information

Calories: 80 Protein: 1g Carbohydrates: 4g Dietary Fiber: 2g Sugar: 1g Fat: 7g

Chia Seed Pudding with Berries

Prep Time: 5 minutes

Servings: 4

Ingredients:

- 1/4 cup of chia seeds
- 1 1/2 cups of unsweetened almond milk
- 1/4 cup of granulated erythritol or monk fruit sweetener
- 1 tsp vanilla extract
- 1/4 tsp sea salt
- 1/2 cup of mixed fresh berries
- 1 tbsp unsweetened shredded coconut
- Fresh mint leaves

Instructions:

1. Combine the chia seeds, almond milk, sweetener, vanilla extract, and sea salt in a medium bowl.
2. Cover the bowl and chill for at least 2 hours, preferably overnight, for the best effects. Stir the mixture after the first 10 minutes to avoid clumping.
3. Mix the chia pudding well when it has thickened to a creamy consistency. If it's too thick, add more almond milk until it reaches the right consistency.
4. Divide the pudding amongst serving bowls or jars. Garnish with fresh berries, shredded coconut, and a sprig of mint.
5. Serve chilled.

Nutrition Information (Per Serving):

Calories: 140 Protein: 4g Carbohydrates: 10g Dietary Fiber: 7g Sugar: 2g Fat: 9g

Keto Almond Butter Fudge

Prep Time: 10 minutes

Servings: 16 squares

Ingredients:

- 1 cup of almond butter
- 1/4 cup of coconut oil, melted
- 1/4 cup of powdered erythritol or monk fruit sweetener
- 1 tsp vanilla extract
- 1/4 tsp sea salt
- 1/4 cup of chopped almonds
- 2 tbsp sugar-free dark chocolate chips

Instructions:

1. Combine almond butter, melted coconut oil, powdered sweetener, vanilla extract, and sea salt in a medium mixing bowl. Stir until smooth and well blended.
2. Add the chopped almonds for added texture.
3. Prepare a small baking dish or loaf pan with parchment paper. Pour the fudge onto the pan and use a spatula to distribute it evenly.
4. Place the pan in the refrigerator for at least 1 hour or until the fudge has set. If desired, melt the sugar-free chocolate chips and sprinkle them on the cold fudge.
5. When the fudge is solid, remove it from the pan using the parchment paper. Cut it into 16 squares, and enjoy.

Nutrition Information (Per Square):

Calories: 120 Protein: 3g Carbohydrates: 4g Dietary Fiber: 2g Sugar: 1g Fat: 11g

Strawberry & Cream Keto Popsicles

Prep Time: 10 minutes

Servings: 6 popsicles

Ingredients:

- 1 1/2 cups of fresh strawberries, hulled
- 1/2 cup of heavy cream
- 1/4 cup of unsweetened almond milk
- 2 tbsp powdered erythritol
- 1 tsp vanilla extract
- 1 tbsp lemon juice

Instructions:

1. Mix the strawberries, heavy cream, almond milk, sweetener, vanilla extract, and lemon juice (if desired) in a blender. Blend until smooth and creamy.
2. Taste the mixture and adjust the sweetness as needed by adding a bit more sweetener.
3. Pour the strawberry mixture equally into the popsicle molds. Tap the molds lightly against the counter to expel any air bubbles.
4. Insert the popsicle sticks and freeze the molds for at least 4 hours or until the popsicles are completely set.
5. To remove the popsicles, run the molds under warm water for a few seconds or gently pull on their sticks.
6. Serve immediately.

Nutrition Information (Per Popsicle):

Calories: 70 Protein: 1g Carbohydrates: 4g Dietary Fiber: 1g Sugar: 2g Fat: 6g

Coconut Flour Brownies

Prep Time: 10 minutes

Cook Time: 20-25 minutes

Servings: 12 brownies

Ingredients:

- 1/4 cup of coconut flour
- 1/2 cup of unsweetened cocoa powder
- 1/2 cup of granulated erythritol
- 1/2 cup of melted coconut oil
- 3 large eggs
- 1/4 cup of unsweetened almond milk
- 1 tsp vanilla extract
- 1/4 tsp sea salt
- 1/2 tsp baking powder
- 1/4 cup of sugar-free dark chocolate chips

Instructions:

1. Preheat the oven to 350° Fahrenheit (175° Celsius). Line an 8x8-inch baking dish with parchment paper or gently oil it.
2. In a medium mixing bowl, combine the coconut flour, cocoa powder, sweetener, sea salt, and baking powder until thoroughly blended.
3. In a separate bowl, mix the melted coconut oil, eggs, almond milk, and vanilla extract until smooth.
4. Gradually incorporate the dry ingredients into the wet liquid, stirring until a thick, homogeneous batter forms.
5. Stir in the sugar-free chocolate chips. Pour the batter into the prepared baking dish and spread evenly with a spatula. Bake for 20-25 minutes or until a toothpick inserted in the middle is mostly clean.
6. Allow the brownies to cool in the pan for at least 15 minutes before cutting them into 12 squares.

Nutrition Information (Per Serving):

Calories: 130 Protein: 3g Carbohydrates: 7g Dietary Fiber: 3g Sugar: 1g Fat: 11g

Lemon Coconut Energy Balls

Prep Time: 10 minutes

Servings: 12 energy balls

Ingredients:

- 1 cup of unsweetened shredded coconut
- 1/2 cup of almond flour
- 2 tbsp coconut oil, melted
- 2 tbsp granulated erythritol
- Zest of 1 lemon
- Juice of 1 lemon
- 1/2 tsp vanilla extract
- 1/4 tsp sea salt

Instructions:

1. Add shredded coconut, almond flour, coconut oil, sweetener, lemon zest, lemon juice, vanilla extract, and sea salt in a medium mixing bowl. Stir well until the mixture comes together.
2. Scoop off 1 tbsp of the mixture and form it into a ball with your palms. Repeat until the entire mixture is utilized (approximately 12 energy balls).
3. Place the lemon coconut balls on a bowl and chill for at least 30 minutes until stiff.
4. Enjoy your energy balls.

Nutrition Information

Calories: 80 Protein: 1g Carbohydrates: 4g Dietary Fiber: 2g Sugar: 1g Fat: 7g

Chocolate Protein Truffles

Prep Time: 10 minutes

Servings: 12 truffles

Ingredients:

- 1/2 cup of unsweetened cocoa powder
- 1/2 cup of almond flour
- 1/4 cup of protein powder
- 1/4 cup of powdered erythritol
- 1/4 cup of coconut oil, melted
- 2 tbsp unsweetened almond milk
- 1 tsp vanilla extract
- Pinch of sea salt
- 1/4 cup of sugar-free dark chocolate chips

Instructions:

1. Add cocoa powder, almond flour, protein powder, sweetener, and a sprinkle of sea salt in a large mixing bowl. Stir well to mix.
2. Combine the melted coconut oil, almond milk, and vanilla extract with the dry ingredients. Stir until a thick and sticky dough forms.
3. Scoop off 1 tbsp of the mixture and form it into a ball with your palms. Repeat until all of the dough is utilized, yielding approximately 12 truffles.
4. Melt the sugar-free dark chocolate chips in the microwave or a double boiler. Dip each truffle in melted chocolate and set on a parchment-lined platter.
5. Put the truffles in the fridge for 30 minutes to harden up. Serve these rich and fudgy chocolate protein truffles chilled.

Nutrition Information

Calories: 90 Protein: 4g Carbohydrates: 5g Dietary Fiber: 3g Sugar: 1g Fat: 7g

Pumpkin Spice Fat Bombs

Prep Time: 10 minutes

Servings: 12 fat bombs

Ingredients:

- 1/2 cup of canned pumpkin puree (unsweetened)
- 1/2 cup of cream cheese, softened
- 1/4 cup of coconut oil, melted
- 1/4 cup of powdered erythritol or monk fruit sweetener
- 1 tsp vanilla extract
- 1 tsp pumpkin pie spice
- 1/4 tsp cinnamon
- Pinch of sea salt

Instructions:

1. Combine the pumpkin puree, cream cheese, and coconut oil in a medium mixing bowl until smooth. Add the sweetener, vanilla extract, pumpkin pie spice, cinnamon, and sea salt and mix until well combined.
2. Divide the mixture into 1-inch balls and set on a parchment-lined dish or baking sheet.
3. Refrigerate the fat bombs for at least 30 minutes or until firm. For a firmer texture, freeze for 15-20 minutes.
4. Once firm, transfer the fat bombs to an airtight jar and refrigerate. Enjoy chilled.

Nutrition Information (Per Fat Bomb):

Calories: 80 Protein: 1g Carbohydrates: 3g Dietary Fiber: 1g Sugar: 1g Fat: 8g

Low-Carb Cinnamon Apple Crisp

Prep Time: 15 minutes Cook Time: 30 minutes Servings: 6

Ingredients:

- 4 medium-sized apples
- 2 tbsp lemon juice
- 1/4 cup of granulated erythritol or monk fruit sweetener
- 1 tsp ground cinnamon
- 1/4 tsp ground nutmeg
- 1/4 tsp ground allspice (optional)
- 1/4 tsp sea salt
- 1 cup of almond flour
- 1/2 cup of chopped pecans (or walnuts)
- 1/4 cup of unsweetened shredded coconut
- 1/4 cup of granulated erythritol or monk fruit sweetener
- 1/4 cup of melted coconut oil (or butter)
- 1 tsp ground cinnamon
- 1/4 tsp sea salt

Instructions:

1. Preheat the oven to 350° Fahrenheit (175° Celsius). Grease an 8x8-inch baking dish with coconut oil or butter.
2. Peel, core, and finely slice your apples. Combine the apple slices, lemon juice, sugar, cinnamon, nutmeg, allspice, and sea salt in a large mixing bowl. Spread the apples equally in the prepared baking dish.
3. In a separate mixing bowl, combine almond flour, chopped nuts, shredded coconut (if using), sweetener, melted coconut oil, cinnamon, and sea salt. Stir until the mixture has a crumbly texture.
4. Sprinkle the crumble topping evenly over the apple mixture.
5. Place the dish in the oven and bake for 25-30 minutes until the apples are soft and the topping is golden brown.
6. Allow the crisp to cool for ten minutes before serving. Enjoy when still warm.

Nutrition Information (Per Serving):

Calories: 180 Protein: 3g Carbohydrates: 10g Dietary Fiber: 4g Sugar: 5g Fat: 14g

Coconut Panna Cotta

Prep Time: 10 minutes

Servings: 4

Ingredients:

- 1 can (14 oz) full-fat coconut milk
- 1/2 cup of unsweetened almond milk
- 1/4 cup of powdered erythritol or monk fruit sweetener
- 1 tsp vanilla extract
- 1 packet (2 tsp) unflavored gelatin
- 2 tbsp cold water
- Pinch of sea salt
- Fresh berries or toasted unsweetened coconut flakes

Instructions:

1. Combine the gelatin and cold water in a small bowl. Allow it to rest for 5 minutes to bloom.
2. Mix the coconut milk, almond milk, sweetener, vanilla extract, and sea salt in a saucepan. Cook over medium heat, stirring often, until the mixture is heated but not boiling.
3. When the milk mixture is heated, remove from the heat and whisk in the bloomed gelatin until thoroughly dissolved.
4. Divide the contents evenly into four small ramekins or dessert glasses.
5. Refrigerate for at least 4 hours or until the panna cotta is solid and stiff.
6. To serve, run a knife along the edge of each ramekin and invert onto a bowl, or serve straight into the dessert glasses. If preferred, top with fresh berries or toasted coconut flakes.

Nutrition Information (Per Serving):

Calories: 160 Protein: 2g Carbohydrates: 4g Dietary Fiber: 1g Sugar: 1g Fat: 15g

Peanut Butter & Chocolate Keto Cup

Prep Time: 15 minutes

Servings: 12 cups

Ingredients:

- For the Chocolate Layer:
- 1/2 cup of sugar-free dark chocolate chips
- 2 tbsp coconut oil
- For the Peanut Butter Layer:
- 1/2 cup of creamy peanut butter
- 2 tbsp coconut oil, melted
- 2 tbsp powdered erythritol
- 1/2 tsp vanilla extract
- Pinch of sea salt

Instructions:

1. In a microwave-safe bowl, melt the sugar-free chocolate chips and coconut oil in 30-second increments, stirring in between, until smooth.
2. Pour approximately 1 tsp of the melted chocolate mixture into each portion of a tiny muffin pan or silicone mold. Tilt the pan to cover the sides in chocolate. Place the pan in the freezer for ten minutes to solidify.
3. Combine peanut butter, heated coconut oil, sweetener, vanilla extract, and sea salt in a separate bowl until smooth.
4. Remove the pan from the freezer. Spread approximately 1 tsp of peanut butter mixture over the firm chocolate layer. Smooth the top using a spoon.
5. Spoon the remaining chocolate mixture evenly over the peanut butter layer, thoroughly covering the top.
6. Return the pan to the freezer for at least 30 minutes or until the cups are hard.
7. Take the cups of out of the molds and enjoy!

Nutrition Information (Per Cup of):

Calories: 130 Protein: 3g Carbohydrates: 5g Dietary Fiber: 2g Sugar: 1g Fat: 12g

Almond Butter Blondies

Prep Time: 10 minutes

Cook Time: 20-25 minutes

Servings: 12 blondies

Ingredients:

- 1 cup of creamy almond butter
- 2 large eggs
- 1/2 cup of granulated erythritol or monk fruit sweetener
- 1/4 cup of almond flour
- 1 tsp vanilla extract
- 1/2 tsp baking powder
- 1/4 tsp sea salt
- 1/4 cup of sugar-free dark chocolate chips

Instructions:

1. Preheat the oven to 350° Fahrenheit (175° Celsius). Line an 8x8-inch baking sheet with parchment paper or gently oil it.
2. Mix almond butter, eggs, and vanilla extract in a large bowl and whisk until creamy.
3. Combine the sweetener, almond flour, baking powder, and sea salt. Mix until well combined. If using sugar-free chocolate chips, fold them in.
4. Pour the batter into the prepared baking pan and spread evenly with a spatula.
5. Place the pan in the preheated oven for 20-25 minutes, or until the rims are golden brown and a toothpick inserted into the middle comes out almost clean.
6. Allow the blondies to cool in the pan for at least 15 minutes before cutting into 12 squares.

Nutrition Information (Per Blondie):

Calories: 160 Protein: 5g Carbohydrates: 6g Dietary Fiber: 3g Sugar: 1g Fat: 14g

Mocha Coconut Keto Ice Cream

Prep Time: 15 minutes

Servings: 6

Ingredients:

- 1 can (14 oz) full-fat coconut milk
- 1/2 cup of heavy cream
- 1/4 cup of unsweetened cocoa powder
- 2 tbsp instant coffee or espresso powder
- 1/3 cup of powdered erythritol or monk fruit sweetener
- 1 tsp vanilla extract
- Pinch of sea salt
- 1/4 cup of sugar-free dark chocolate chips (optional)
- 1/4 cup of unsweetened shredded coconut (optional)

Instructions:

1. In a medium mixing bowl, blend the coconut milk, heavy cream, cocoa powder, instant coffee, sweetener, vanilla extract, and sea salt until thoroughly combined. Make sure there are no lumps of cocoa powder or coffee.
2. Cover the bowl and chill the mixture for at least 1-2 hours to allow the flavors to combine.
3. Pour the cold ingredients into an ice cream maker and churn according to the manufacturer's directions. If you don't own an ice cream machine, check the note below for a no-churn alternative.
4. Incorporate sugar-free chocolate chips in the final 5 minutes of churning.
5. Transfer the ice cream to an airtight jar and freeze for 2-3 hours for a firmer texture.
6. Scoop the ice cream into bowls, then sprinkle with unsweetened shredded coconut if preferred. Enjoy!

Nutrition Information (Per Serving):

Calories: 180 Protein: 2g Carbohydrates: 6g Dietary Fiber: 3g Sugar: 1g Fat: 16g

30 DAYS MEAL PLAN

Day	Breakfast	Lunch	Dinner	Snack/Dessert
01	Avocado & Spinach Power Omelet	Grilled Chicken & Quinoa Salad	Baked Salmon with Asparagus	Guacamole & Veggie Sticks
02	Greek Yogurt Parfait with Nuts & Berries	Cauliflower Rice Stir-Fry with Shrimp	Garlic & Herb Roasted Chicken with Brussels Sprouts	Keto Vanilla Mug Cake
03	Almond Butter & Chia Seed Smoothie	Zucchini Noodles with Pesto & Cherry Tomatoes	Zucchini Lasagna with Ground Turkey	Deviled Eggs with Avocado
04	Protein Pancakes with Fresh Berries	Spinach & Avocado Tuna Salad	Beef & Broccoli Stir-Fry	Lemon & Garlic Roasted Asparagus
05	Cottage Cheese & Cucumber Bowl	Thai Chicken Lettuce Cups	Spaghetti Squash Bolognese	Chocolate Avocado Mousse
06	Coconut Flour Waffles	Turkey & Veggie Lettuce Wraps	Low-Carb Pork Chops with Garlic Mushrooms	Almond-Crusted Mozzarella Sticks
07	Low-Carb Egg Muffins with Veggies	Blackened Shrimp & Cauliflower Grits	Seared Scallops with Zoodles	Strawberry & Cream Keto Popsicles
08	Mushroom & Spinach Breakfast Casserole	Mediterranean Veggie Bowl with Hummus	Grilled Shrimp with Cilantro Lime Cauliflower Rice	Keto-Friendly Trail Mix
09	Keto Cinnamon Chia Pudding	Sesame Salmon Salad	Eggplant Parmesan Casserole	Coconut Flour Brownies
10	Zucchini & Bell Pepper Breakfast Hash	Quinoa & Roasted Veggie Buddha Bowl	Thai Basil Chicken Stir-Fry	Broccoli Cheddar Bites
11	Green Detox Smoothie	Greek Chicken Salad Wrap	Low-Carb Lamb & Vegetable Curry	Lemon Coconut Energy Balls
12	Cottage Cheese & Cucumber Bowl	Chicken Caesar Salad with Kale	Lemon Pepper Tilapia with Steamed Greens	Chocolate Protein Truffles
13	Low-Carb Banana Protein Muffins	Asian Ginger Chicken & Cabbage Slaw	Spicy Cauliflower & Chicken Skillet	Peanut Butter & Chocolate Keto Cups
14	Scrambled Eggs with Kale & Cherry Tomatoes	Turkey & Veggie Lettuce Wraps	Slow-Cooked Beef Stew with Veggies	Cucumber & Avocado Rolls
15	Almond Butter & Chia Seed Smoothie	Zucchini Noodles with Pesto & Cherry Tomatoes	Sheet Pan Salmon & Veggies	Keto Lemon Bars
16	Coconut Flour Waffles	Grilled Halloumi & Arugula Salad	Baked Lemon Herb Cod with Spinach	Cashew Coconut Bark
17	Veggie & Turkey Breakfast Wrap	Low-Carb Taco Salad	Keto-Friendly Stuffed Bell Peppers	Pumpkin Spice Fat Bombs

18	Zucchini & Bell Pepper Breakfast Hash	Spinach & Avocado Tuna Salad	Spaghetti Squash Bolognese	Greek Yogurt Ranch Dip with Cucumbers
19	Cottage Cheese & Cucumber Bowl	Blackened Shrimp & Cauliflower Grits	Grilled Veggie & Chicken Kebabs	Matcha Coconut Balls
20	Low-Carb Egg Muffins with Veggies	Greek Chicken Salad Wrap	Low-Carb Turkey Meatloaf	No-Bake Raspberry Cheesecake Bars
21	Mushroom & Spinach Breakfast Casserole	Cauliflower Rice Stir-Fry with Shrimp	Moroccan-Spiced Chicken with Spinach	Almond Butter Blondies
22	Keto Cinnamon Chia Pudding	Quinoa & Roasted Veggie Buddha Bowl	Thai Basil Chicken Stir-Fry	Low-Carb Cinnamon Apple Crisp
23	Green Detox Smoothie	Turkey & Veggie Lettuce Wraps	Spicy Cauliflower & Chicken Skillet	Vanilla Chia Pudding with Almond Butter Drizzle
24	Protein Pancakes with Fresh Berries	Steak & Roasted Veggie Bowl	Cauliflower Crust Margherita Pizza	Blueberry Coconut Muffins
25	Greek Yogurt Parfait with Nuts & Berries	Lemon Garlic Zoodles with Shredded Chicken	Seared Scallops with Zoodles	Mini Caprese Salad Skewers
26	Almond Butter & Chia Seed Smoothie	Zucchini Noodles with Pesto & Cherry Tomatoes	Low-Carb Lamb & Vegetable Curry	Keto-Friendly Trail Mix
27	Cottage Cheese & Cucumber Bowl	Low-Carb Taco Salad	Moroccan-Spiced Chicken with Spinach	Chocolate Zucchini Bread
28	Scrambled Eggs with Kale & Cherry Tomatoes	Spinach & Avocado Tuna Salad	Beef & Broccoli Stir-Fry	Mocha Coconut Keto Ice Cream
29	Zucchini & Bell Pepper Breakfast Hash	Grilled Chicken & Quinoa Salad	Lemon Pepper Tilapia with Steamed Greens	Coconut Panna Cotta
30	Green Detox Smoothie	Turkey & Veggie Lettuce Wraps	Baked Salmon with Asparagus	Chocolate Avocado Mousse

www.ingramcontent.com/pod-product-compliance
Lightning Source LLC
Chambersburg PA
CBHW082250220526
45469CB00009B/2946